# Nerve Problems of the Lower Extremity

*Guest Editor*

JOHN S. GOULD, MD

# FOOT AND ANKLE CLINICS

www.foot.theclinics.com

*Consulting Editor*
MARK S. MYERSON, MD

June 2011 • Volume 16 • Number 2

SAUNDERS an imprint of ELSEVIER, Inc.

**W.B. SAUNDERS COMPANY**
*A Division of Elsevier Inc.*

1600 John F. Kennedy Blvd. ● Suite 1800 ● Philadelphia, PA 19103-2899

http://www.theclinics.com

**FOOT AND ANKLE CLINICS Volume 16, Number 2**
**June 2011 ISSN 1083-7515, ISBN-13: 978-1-4557-0446-0**

Editor: Debora Dellapena
Developmental Editor: Donald E. Mumford

*Foot and Ankle Clinics* (ISSN 1083-7515) is published quarterly by Elsevier, Inc., 360 Park Avenue South, New York, NY 10010-1710. Months of issue are March, June, September, and December. Periodicals postage paid at New York, NY, and additional mailing offices. Subscription price per year is $271.00 (US individuals), $357.00 (US institutions), $134.00 (US students), $308.00 (Canadian individuals), $422.00 (Canadian institutions), $184.00 (Canadian students), $397.00 (foreign individuals), $422.00 (foreign institutions), and $184.00 (foreign students). To receive student/resident rate, orders must be accompanied by name of affiliated institution, date of term, and the *signature* of program/residency coordinator on institution letterhead. Orders will be billed at individual rate until proof of status is received. Foreign air speed delivery is included in all *Clinics* subscription prices. All prices are subject to change without notice. **POSTMASTER:** Send address changes to *Foot and Ankle Clinics*, Elsevier Health Sciences Division, Subscription Customer Service, 3251 Riverport Lane, Maryland Heights, MO 63043. **Customer Service: 1-800-654-2452 (US and Canada). From outside of the United States and Canada, call 314-447-8871. Fax: 314-447-8029. E-mail: JournalsCustomerService-usa@ elsevier.com (for print support); JournalsOnlineSupport-usa@elsevier.com (for online support).**

*Reprints.* For copies of 100 or more, of articles in this publication, please contact the Commercial Reprints Department, Elsevier Inc., 360 Park Avenue South, New York, NY 10010-1710. Tel.: 212-633-3812; Fax: 212-462-1935; E-mail: reprints@elsevier.com.

Printed and bound by CPI Group (UK) Ltd, Croydon, CR0 4YY

Transferred to Digital Print 2011

# Contributors

## CONSULTING EDITOR

**MARK S. MYERSON, MD**
Director, Institute for Foot and Ankle Reconstruction at Mercy, Mercy Medical Center, Baltimore, Maryland

## GUEST EDITOR

**JOHN S. GOULD, MD**
Chief, Section of Foot and Ankle, University of Alabama at Birmingham, Birmingham; Professor of Surgery, Division of Orthopaedic Surgery; Adjunct Professor of Orthopaedic Surgery, University of South Alabama, Mobile, Alabama

## AUTHORS

**SAMUEL B. ADAMS Jr, MD**
Fellow, Department of Orthopaedic Surgery, Foot and Ankle Service, Union Memorial Hospital, Baltimore, Maryland

**NILESH M. CHAUDHARI, MD**
Assistant Professor of Surgery, Division of Orthopaedic Surgery, Section of Foot and Ankle, University of Alabama at Birmingham, Birmingham, Alabama

**BENEDICT F. DIGIOVANNI, MD**
Associate Professor, Department of Orthopaedics, University of Rochester Medical Center, Rochester, New York

**RYAN M. FLANIGAN, MD**
Resident, Department of Orthopaedics, University of Rochester Medical Center, Rochester, New York

**JOHN S. GOULD, MD**
Chief, Section of Foot and Ankle, University of Alabama at Birmingham, Birmingham; Professor of Surgery, Division of Orthopaedic Surgery; Adjunct Professor of Orthopaedic Surgery, University of South Alabama, Mobile, Alabama

**JOHN S. KIRCHNER, MD**
Assistant Professor of Surgery, Section of Foot and Ankle, Division of Orthopaedic Surgery, University of Alabama at Birmingham, Birmingham, Alabama

**ROBERT LOPEZ-BEN, MD**
Staff Radiologist, Charlotte Radiology, Charlotte, North Carolina

**SUSAN E. MACKINNON, MD**
Division of Plastic and Reconstructive Surgery, Washington University School of Medicine, St Louis, Missouri

**VICTORIA R. MASEAR, MD**
Orthopaedic Specialists of Alabama, Birmingham, Alabama

**CRISTIAN ORTIZ, MD**
Chief, Foot and Ankle Service, Clinica Alemana, Vitacura, Santiago, Chile;
Associate Professor, Universidad del Desarrollo, Escuela de Medicina, Las Condes

**PAUL G. PETERS, MD**
Fellow, Department of Orthopaedic Surgery, Foot and Ankle Service, Union Memorial
Hospital, Baltimore, Maryland

**MICHAEL S. PINZUR, MD**
Professor of Orthopaedic Surgery, Loyola University Health System, Maywood, Illinois

**WILSON Z. RAY, MD**
Department of Neurological Surgery, Washington University School of Medicine,
St Louis, Missouri

**PAIGE C. ROY, MD**
EMG Director and Assistant Professor, Department of Physical Medicine and
Rehabilitation, The University of Alabama at Birmingham, Birmingham, Alabama

**LEW C. SCHON, MD**
Chief of Foot and Ankle Surgery, Department of Orthopaedic Surgery, Foot and Ankle
Service, Union Memorial Hospital, Baltimore, Maryland

**ASHISH SHAH, MD**
Assistant Professor of Surgery, Section of Foot and Ankle, Division of Orthopaedic
Surgery, University of Alabama at Birmingham, Birmingham, Alabama

**EMILIO WAGNER, MD**
Chief, Foot and Ankle Service, Hospital Padre Hurtado, San Ramon; Associate Professor,
Universidad del Desarrollo, Escuela de Medicina, Las Condes; Foot and Ankle Service,
Clinica Alemana, Vitacura, Santiago, Chile

# Contents

along with the anatomic variation that exists between individuals. Precise knowledge of the anatomic course, the common motor and sensory distributions of each of the peripheral nerves, and judicious use of imaging or electrodiagnostic testing can greatly assist in arriving at a correct diagnosis. In this article, we discuss in detail the anatomy, clinical presentation, diagnosis, and treatment options for peripheral nerve entrapments of the lower extremity involving the sural, saphenous and common, superficial, and deep peroneal nerves.

Tarsal tunnel syndrome, unlike its similar sounding counterpart in the hand, is a significantly misunderstood clinical entity. Confusion concerning the anatomy involved, the presenting symptomatology, the appropriateness and significance of various diagnostic tests, conservative and surgical management, and, finally, the variability of reported results of surgical intervention attests to the lack of consensus surrounding this condition. The terminology involved in various diagnoses for chronic heel pain is also a hodgepodge of poorly understood entities.

Failed surgical releases of the tarsal tunnel may be due to numerous causes. Many of the failures are due to lack of appreciation of the involved anatomy or inadequate technique. When an insufficient release is done, a revision simply completes the necessary steps. When external scarring is the problem, barrier materials may be used to help protect the nerve after neurolysis. When intrinsic damage is the problem, nerve wrapping, reconstruction, conduits, and nerve stimulators all play a role to restore function or ameliorate pain.

Treatment of neuromas in the foot and ankle is evolving. A paucity of studies deals with neuromas in this region; most knowledge comes from hand surgery. A trend toward reconstructive surgery using nerve grafts and conduits for nerves with critical function is being seen. For noncritical nerves, generally accepted treatment is neuroma resection and burial into a tissue bed. A clear knowledge of neural anatomy is paramount, together with correct identification of all the nerves involved in the pain-generation process. More studies dealing with neuromas in this area are needed for evidence-based information.

Interdigital neuralgia affects a significant number of individuals, with an average age of presentation in the sixth decade and a 4- to 15-fold increased prevalence in women. Historical descriptions date back to the 19th century. Nonoperative treatment with shoe modifications, metatarsal pads, and injections provides relief for most, but long term, 60% to 70% of patients eventually elect to have surgery. Although excision can be performed through a dorsal or plantar approach, we prefer the dorsal incision to prevent scar formation on the plantar aspect of the foot. Satisfactory results are common but not certain with reports of excellent or good ranging from 51% to 93%.

Recurrent or persistent symptoms following surgical neurectomy for an interdigital neuroma are quite common, because of incorrect initial diagnosis, true neuroma formation, nerve stump adhesions, accessory nerve branches, or an adjacent web space neuroma. The clinical presentation of a recurrent neuroma is similar to the initial presentation. Recurrent symptoms usually occur within the first 12 months after surgery. The physical examination coupled with diagnostic nerve blocks is critical for diagnosis. Conservative therapy, although not particularly effective in treating true recurrent neuromas, may help to alleviate pain. With proper isolation of the instigating neuroma, revision surgical excision can be effective.

Nerve scarring can cause severe pain and dysfunction. Treatment of the scarred nerve frequently yields unpredictable results. A barrier wrap around the scarred nerve could be of benefit in preventing the recurrence of epineural scarring following neurolysis. The barrier would ideally be inert so as to not incite an inflammatory response, and be nondegradable. Veins fulfill both of these objectives. The desirable qualities of a barrier nerve wrap include a substance that decreases nerve scarring, does not constrict and thus compress the nerve, and improves nerve gliding. The primary indication for nerve wrapping is a nerve with adherent scar.

Treatment of the chronic painful nerve by pedicled or free tissue transfer is a complex surgical procedure, requiring specialized microsurgical training and technique. This procedure is indicated only in patients who have had repeated failure of simpler, conventional procedures. Patients with chronic painful peripheral nerves may be potentially salvaged by external neurolysis and circumferential wrapping of the involved segments of nerve with well-vascularized pedicled or free flaps of fascia, subcutaneous fatty tissue, omentum or muscle, or by the replacement of superficial hypersensitive cutaneous areas and nerves with the same tissues.

Diabetic peripheral neuropathy likely affects up to one-third of adults with diabetes. All diabetic patients are likely to develop peripheral neuropathy if they live sufficiently long. Recognition is crucial for initiation of the preventive strategies that have been demonstrated to decrease the potential risk for the development of diabetic foot ulcers, foot infection, Charcot foot, or amputation. The mainstay of current treatment is optimal glucose and hemoglobin $A_{1C}$ control. Drug therapy has limited potential for controlling the associated pain. Alternative methods of treatment have thus far demonstrated limited success.

Complex regional pain syndrome (CRPS) is a challenging pain condition for doctors and patients, with a natural history characterized by chronicity and relapses that can result in significant disability. CRPS is difficult to diagnose and treat, and requires close follow-up to ensure that progress is being made. Early diagnosis and treatment are required to prevent a long-standing or permanent disability. Clinical features such as spontaneous pain, edema, hyperalgesia, temperature or sudomotor changes, motor function abnormality, and autonomic changes are the hallmark of this disease. The treatment of CRPS remains controversial, and includes medications, physical therapy, regional anesthesia, and neuromodulation.

**THE CLINICS ARE NOW AVAILABLE ONLINE!**

Access your subscription at:
**www.theclinics.com**

# Preface

# Nerve Problems of the Lower Extremity

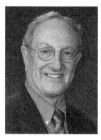

John S. Gould, MD
*Guest Editor*

This issue on Nerve Problems of the Lower Extremity, which focuses primarily on the foot and ankle, is an update on the latest approaches to the diagnosis and management of the nerve disorders that we as orthopedic specialists in the foot and ankle encounter in our academic and private practices.

The articles on imaging and electrodiagnostic evaluations contain new ideas on objective ways to diagnose and document many conditions that just a few years ago could only be diagnosed by the astute clinician with his history and physical examination. The importance of the latter is still emphasized.

The article by MacKinnon and Ray discusses the latest concepts in repair and reconstruction, while entrapments by Flanagan and DiGiovanni update our understanding of these frequent conditions. Management of neuromas, interdigital neuromas and recurrences, and tarsal tunnel and failed tarsal tunnel release are covered by acknowledged experts who submit, albeit with bias, their approaches to these difficult entities.

The current status of nerve wrapping techniques and results, flap coverage for painful nerves, and updates on diabetic neuropathy and complex regional pain syndromes completes the volume.

This publication does not presume to be comprehensive and the approaches described are a compilation of "expert opinion" rather than a synopsis of the current literature. Review journals are available to provide such information. These articles not only reflect the bias of the authors, but also of the editor, and my selection of particular authors to write the articles. I admit this and apologize if alternative approaches have not always been forthcoming. Nonetheless, I believe the readers of the volume will be interested and even fascinated, at times, to read the opinions

Foot Ankle Clin N Am 16 (2011) xi–xii
doi:10.1016/j.fcl.2011.04.002
1083-7515/11/$ – see front matter © 2011 Elsevier Inc. All rights reserved.

of these well-known authors and that the material presented will at least be provocative and stimulating.

John S. Gould, MD
Section of Foot and Ankle
Division of Orthopaedic Surgery
University of Alabama at Birmingham
1313 13th Street, South #226
Birmingham, AL 35205, USA

E-mail address:
Gouldjs@aol.com

# Clinical Evaluation of Neurogenic Conditions

Neurogenic problems of the foot and ankle are far more common than often appreciated. From well-known conditions such as Morton neuroma and tarsal tunnel syndrome to peripheral neuropathy, the foot is a frequent target for issues related to the peripheral nervous system, as well as those of the central nervous system. This issue of *Foot and Ankle Clinics of North America* does not deal with the central nervous system and the manifestations of stroke, cerebral palsy, muscular dystrophy, Parkinson disease, or multiple sclerosis, but it should be noted that orthopedic foot and ankle surgeons must be cognizant of how to diagnose and treat them, as well as the roles of medication, physical medicine, rehabilitation, orthotics, and the use of judicious surgery in the care of these patients.

As diagnosticians, we must also be able to differentiate among peripheral neuropathy, radiculopathy, and distal lesions directly involving the peripheral nerves. The initial challenge is to determine that the source of pain or dysfunction is indeed nervous in origin, then to determine the site of the lesion, and finally to know the options for treatment, nonoperative and surgical. Indications for surgery and the best methods for restoring function and relieving pain are also required components of the surgeon's armamentarium.

## DIAGNOSIS

Making the diagnosis may not be easy, as objective modalities such as radiography or computed tomography (CT) are frequently not helpful and magnetic resonance imaging (MRI) may be misleading. The most essential element in making a diagnosis is the history. The art of history taking is often challenging in the case of nerve disorders. A rambling discourse by the patient on the circumstances related to the problem is usually not particularly helpful, including a litany of the many doctors and paramedical personnel they have seen and the various modalities that have been attempted empirically. Nevertheless, this "saga" of attempted medical treatment efforts and the accompanying travelogue indicate that the problem *is* difficult and *could be* neurogenic. Clues such as "no improvement, even worse after casting or other forms of immobilization" or increased pain after attempted physical therapy, especially with the application of heat, cold, or vibration, also suggests a neurogenic cause.

The objective of the history is to determine or rule out a mechanical cause or to sort out various other types of nonmechanical diagnoses. It is also important to remember pseudomechanical factors ("the longer I stand or walk, the worse the symptoms become"), which can be primarily neurogenic, as well as mechanical issues such as an arthritic joint or inflamed swollen tendon sheath, which can irritate an adjacent or overlying nerve. Here, the patient may present with both arthritic and neurogenic symptoms. It should also be noted that tenosynovitis and bursitis may radiate and burn as well as irritate the nerves.

Classically, neurogenic symptoms include pain (aching, burning, itching, stabbing), paresthesias, numbness, autonomic complaints (sweating, dryness), and motor

Foot Ankle Clin N Am 16 (2011) xiii–xvi
doi:10.1016/j.fcl.2011.01.007
1083-7515/11/$ – see front matter © 2011 Elsevier Inc. All rights reserved.

weakness and paralysis. These complaints may be intermittent, continuous, occurring at rest, and frequently occurring at night or awaking a person from sleep. As noted earlier, these symptoms may be aggravated by activity. However, it is important to note that all these symptoms do not have to be present when the cause is neurogenic. For example, in many cases of mechanical causes, pain stops with rest or sitting down and, in some, almost immediately, whereas an afterburn or continuing pain after the cessation of activity may be the only clue for a neurogenic cause.

### History Taking

I always begin by asking about the circumstances surrounding the initial symptoms. A crush injury without the occurrence of the fracture, which continues to be painful, especially with subsequent immobilization for a period beyond the time for a subtle fracture to be healed, suggests injury to a superficial nerve such as the superficial peroneal. An inversion injury with persistent symptoms along the course of the same nerve suggests a traction or stretch injury. Pain at rest suggests oncologic, infectious, or neurogenic causes. To sort this out, I need to probe further about the time of the symptom occurrence. After asking about the original circumstances surrounding the onset of symptoms, I ask if the patient has these symptoms before getting out of bed in the morning, if pain or the other symptoms occur with the first step in the morning (suggesting enthesopathies), if pain disappears after a few steps or gets worse with ambulation (as in a nerve entrapment or other causes of a mechanical nature), and then the critical question of whether it is relieved by sitting down, as noted earlier. Specifically, "How quickly does the pain or other symptoms go away?" Further questions can help rule out infectious causes in most instances, particularly if there is no site of entry for an organism or other systemic symptoms, such as a urinary tract infection or an oral or upper respiratory tract infection that could account for a hematogenous transmission of such an infection.

Many patients report that their pain, for instance, radiates from their foot up the back of the leg to their back, which can usually be translated to actually occur in the reverse direction. Questions concerning their back should be asked, and the back should subsequently be tested in the physical examination. When attempting to determine if generalized neuropathy should be considered, bilaterality, as well as ascending symptoms, is usually reported. Although electrodiagnostic studies should be conclusive for this diagnosis, the cause depends on the history. Alcoholism, hyperthyroidism, and diabetes mellitus are the main causes in this country, along with radiation and heavy metal poisoning, and a myriad of other causes internationally. What I have found particularly interesting is the finding of classic neuropathy in patients who deny the possibility of diabetes and have normal blood sugar and other hematologic test results but a strong family history of the disease. When the patient's siblings and a parent have manifested diabetes, it seems clear that neuropathy in this patient is a manifestation of a complex disease whose genetic pattern still needs further study.

Although patients may wish to tell you more about what each of their medical care givers may have said about their diagnosis, it is essential that you get the answers to the crucial questions as noted. A careful, probing history is invaluable in sorting out the category of the diagnosis.

### Physical Examination

Knowledge of precise surface anatomy is essential and is the hallmark of a good orthopedic surgeon's examination. The orthopedic surgeon can place his or her finger on the exact location of every bone, joint, tendon, and nerve in the foot and ankle. Although some compulsive patients mark on their skin sites of tenderness or pain or attempt to move the examiner's finger to "where it hurts," it behooves the surgeon to palpate the potential anatomic sites of pathology to see if that location is tender or not. The examination also includes the usual ranges of motion, movements that increase the pain or other symptoms, and the appearance of the patient while standing and walking facing the examiner and from the sagittal and posterior perspectives. When entrapment or injury is suspected, potential sites for the phenomenon should be palpated or lightly percussed for tenderness or paresthesias. When dealing with a nerve laceration or repair, loss of function, motor, sensory, and autonomic, should be tested. In addition, the proximal and distal Tinel sign should be marked on the extremity, and the distance between the two measured to determine the extent of regeneration, if present. Active ranges of motions, motion against resistance while palpating a specific tendon or muscle, and manual motor testing are all part of the neurologic examination. Observation for atrophy or simple stroking of a digit for autonomic changes (smoothness, lack of rugal pattern, or loss of sweating) helps with the diagnosis. Simple testing aids such as the Semmes-Weinstein monofilaments, the starch iodine test for sweating, or even the inflation of a tourniquet to induce nerve pain caused by increased sensitivity to ischemia may help define the diagnosis and localize the lesion.

## CORRELATING THE HISTORY AND THE PHYSICAL EXAMINATION

Correlating the information obtained from the history and the physical examination is the next level of the diagnostic effort. If the components are compatible, you know that you are on the right track. You know the nature of the problem and the site of the lesion. In addition, you may need to add other information. For example, you may have decided that the problem is neurogenic, but the patient's tenderness is in multiple locations. This finding requires the knowledge of how certain lesions typically present and to correlate your findings with this information. A simple example is that a patient may have a tender arthritic joint and an irritated nerve coursing over it. But a little more complicated issue is to know that in tarsal tunnel syndrome, the patient complains of pain in the heel, the longitudinal arch, and the posteromedial ankle. On examination, however, tenderness is found over the posteromedial "soft spot" (see article on tarsal tunnel by John S. Gould elsewhere in this issue for further exploration of this topic), the tibial nerve on the posteromedial ankle, *and* in all the intermetatarsal spaces and webs, distally. This does not mean that the patient has primary pathology in the intermetatarsal nerves (such as a Morton neuroma) as well or a "double crush." The nerve and its branches are simply all hypersensitive. In the latter condition of primary pathology in the intermetatarsal nerve level, the complaint is of metatarsalgia, not heel pain, even though the tibial nerve may also be tender at the posteromedial soft spot, proximally. This understanding is essential in collating the history and physical examination and making the correct diagnosis. At times, the history and physical findings are not compatible at all. Although this can be a reflection of a gap in history taking or a lack of the examiner's knowledge or experience, it is also an ominous sign of psychogenic causes or malingering. Do not make a definitive diagnosis when the history and the physical findings are not compatible.

### Additional Testing

The worst errors in diagnosis are made when findings on auxiliary tests do not fit with the history and the physical examination findings. These errors occur when radiological reports are taken out of context or the radiologist's differential diagnosis, even when incompatible with the history and physical examination findings, is taken as a definitive answer to a long-awaited diagnosis. A recent patient of mine was given a full course of intravenous antibiotic therapy for osteomyelitis of the os calcis based on a report of signal changes on an MRI, which read, "cannot rule out osteomyelitis." A year later, when she first presented to me, she complained that she now had osteomyelitis on the other heel. She had osteoporosis, pain and tenderness of the heel, and signal changes on the MRI. As she had obtained her MRI elsewhere and was certain of her diagnosis, which previously had been treated successfully, she wanted intravenous antibiotics. There was no history of infection elsewhere in the body and no history of trauma to the area. With her recent MRI done and requested elsewhere, her insurance company would not certify my request for a CT scan. A request for an ultrasound-guided aspiration of the bone was granted, and the results revealed and confirmed my suspicion of a stress fracture, which I was sure was the diagnosis on the contralateral heel as well. She was treated successfully without further antibiotics. Another patient with a vague history of ankle and hindfoot pain was referred by an internist, when a radiograph revealed an old, totally asymptomatic great toe interphalangeal joint fracture. The patient had no complaints in that area and no swelling or tenderness.

Radiographs, of course, are essential to rule out various conditions; a CT scan is critical for detailed information about bones and joints but should not be used as a screening tool. The MRI can be helpful as well, but these tests should not be ordered unless there is evidence on the history and physical examination to suggest the need for them. The articles on imaging and electrodiagnosis explain the indications and limits of these studies and how they can help delineate, clarify, and document a diagnosis (see articles by Lopez-Ben; and Paige C. Roy elsewhere in this issue for further exploration of this topic). The electrical studies are essential in radiculopathy, generalized neuropathy, and in severe entrapment and traumatic lesions of peripheral nerves. MRI may also document the sites of trauma, and with high resolution, closely spaced imaging, sites of entrapment may be seen or highly suspected. Ultrasonography has been very useful when done by experienced ultrasonographers.

## SUMMARY

Making the diagnosis of a neurogenic etiology primarily requires good history taking and physical examination. The judicious and appropriate use of electrodiagnostic and imaging studies help clarify and document the diagnosis, but are not substitutes for the basic elements needed to determine the cause and exact location of the patient's problem.

John S. Gould, MD
Section of Foot and Ankle
Division of Orthopaedic Surgery
University of Alabama at Birmingham
1313 13th Street, South #226
Birmingham, AL 35205, USA

E-mail address:
Gouldjs@aol.com

# Imaging of Nerve Entrapment in the Foot and Ankle

Robert Lopez-Ben, MD

**KEYWORDS**

• Nerve entrapment • Foot • Ankle • Imaging

Neuropathies can be a cause of chronic foot and ankle pain. The diagnosis can be elusive given the sometimes nonspecific clinical presentation. Although electrodiagnostic studies are primarily relied on for the diagnosis of nerve impairment, imaging is sometimes helpful in helping define the exact site of the entrapment and whether any masses are present. It is critical for the imager to understand the complex anatomy of these nerves and their adjacent structures, to know the most common locations for their entrapments or injury, and to select the proper imaging modality to improve detection of these difficult-to-diagnose clinical conditions.

Cross-sectional imaging of the peripheral nerves of the foot and ankle is primarily accomplished with ultrasound (US) and magnetic resonance imaging (MRI). Interpretation and performance of these studies can be challenging because of the small caliber of these nerves as well as their variable courses. However, improvements in imaging technologies for both US and MRI have increased diagnostic confidence in the imaging of peripheral nerves in the extremities. Specifically, the availability of high-frequency linear US transducers in ranges of 10 MHz and greater, as well as the development of improved MRI coils and the use of 3 Tesla (T) magnets with their increased signal/noise ratios, have made a large difference in small body part imaging.

The selection of either modality depends on the training and confidence of the imager with each, but, in many cases, they are complementary and it behooves the imager to become confident and adept at both modalities. MRI is unsurpassed in the breadth of the spectrum it can provide by imaging not only the soft tissues but also the osseous components. US is limited to the soft tissues and dependent on the operator's knowledge of anatomy and technical expertise with the transducer. In addition, its spatial resolution can be as much as an order of magnitude greater than MRI with currently available imaging coils.

MRI of the foot and ankle can directly visualize small nerves if careful attention is given to technique for increasing spatial resolution. The use of an increased number of excitations (NEX) or higher field magnets, such as 3 T systems, and dedicated

---

Charlotte Radiology, 1701 East Boulevard, Charlotte, NC 28203, USA
*E-mail address:* bobrlopez@gmail.com

Foot Ankle Clin N Am 16 (2011) 213–224
doi:10.1016/j.fcl.2011.04.001
1083-7515/11/$ – see front matter © 2011 Elsevier Inc. All rights reserved.

foot and ankle phased array MRI coils, increases available signal and allows for larger matrix sizes and decreased pixel size, with consequent decrease in volume averaging.[1] Entrapped nerves show characteristic findings, including increased T2 signal, loss of fascicular pattern, diffuse enlargement, as well as focal swelling.[2–5]

MRI denervation changes in the muscles (increased muscle signal or edema on T2 initially, followed by fatty infiltration and volume loss, best seen on T1 images, with more chronicity of denervation) enervated by a specific nerve, are a sensitive indirect finding of nerve impairment (**Figs. 1** and **2**). This finding of initially increased T2 signal is considered to be secondary to enlargement of the intramuscular capillary bed, which leads to an increase in intramuscular blood volume and extracellular fluid.[6] The anatomic pattern of muscle edema distribution should be specific to those supplied by the affected nerve.

However, in the foot, this may not be as useful, because most of the distal nerves in the foot are predominantly sensory. Also, muscle edema on MRI has an extensive differential diagnosis, including infection, inflammatory myositis, and sequelae of trauma. Because distal nerve branching variations are common in the feet, attempting to determine specific patterns of nerve involvement by distribution of muscle denervation patterns may also prove difficult. Distinguishing small sensory nerves from adjacent vessels can also be difficult with non–contrast-enhanced MRI.[7]

Compared with standard 1.5-T MRI with commercially available receiver coils used most frequently in routine clinical practice, US has improved spatial resolution, allowing for greater detail of the nerve fascicles.[8] Focal swelling of the nerve can be easily detected, and, given the nature of US, direct visualization of the nerve with correlation with symptoms, and with overlying transducer pressure, is helpful in identifying the sites of abnormality. Superficial nerves can be followed easily in cross section through their courses through the ankle and foot by using high-resolution linear transducers, preferably with frequencies greater than 10 MHz (**Fig. 3**), which is in contrast with MRI: the fixed prescribed imaging planes in MRI lead to artifacts of some of these small nerves as they traverse in and out of the imaging plane. However, visualization with US can sometimes be difficult in the plantar aspect of the foot because the nerves dive deep into the plantar intrinsic foot muscles, or if the patient has marked keratosis of the soles of the foot.[7]

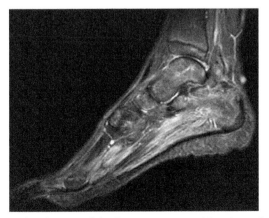

**Fig. 1.** Sagittal T2-weighted image of the foot in a 12-year-old patient who underwent prior resection of a synovial sarcoma with secondary posterior tibial nerve dysfunction. There is increased T2 signal in the intrinsic plantar muscles of the foot from denervation (muscle edema).

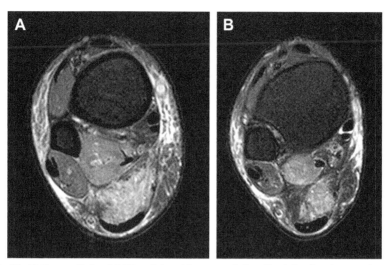

**Fig. 2.** (*A, B*) Sequential axial T2-weighted images of the distal foreleg in a patient with prior crush injury to the tibial nerve, showing denervation muscle edema of the distal soleus and the posterior tibial muscles, which are innervated by the posterior tibial nerve. Note the normal muscle signal in the peroneus brevis muscle laterally and the visualized distal extensor digitorum longus muscle anteriorly; these muscles are not innervated by the tibial nerve.

US can also be used to direct diagnostic and therapeutic nerve injections with improved efficacy, decrease procedure time, and possibly increase the duration of effect compared with traditional surface landmarks or electrical neurostimulation methods of nerve localization.[9–11] The area of focal swelling, or immediately proximal to it, can be targeted with direct real-time US visualization and injection of 2 to 4 mL of local anesthetic (0.25% bupivacaine in our practice) and/or a mixture of local anesthetic and corticosteroid around the nerve, performed with the usual aseptic technique after careful prepping and draping.

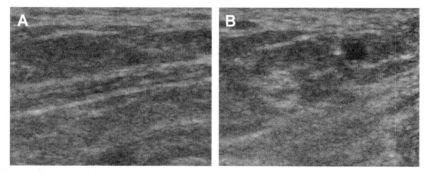

**Fig. 3.** (*A*) Longitudinal US image of a normal-appearing sural nerve. The perineurium has increased echogenicity, as well as the epineurium, which accounts for the intrinsic linear echogenic areas within the nerve that shows normal size and contour as it courses next to the Achilles within the subcutaneous fat. (*B*) Transverse US image of a normal-appearing sural nerve. The lesser saphenous vein is the tubular hypoechoic structure to the right of the nerve, which is the small rounded hyperechoic structure.

Specific nerves in the lower extremity to be evaluated with imaging include the posterior tibial nerve and its main branches, including medial and lateral plantar nerves and inferior calcaneal nerve; the superficial and deep peroneal nerves; and the sural and saphenous nerves.

## POSTERIOR TIBIAL NERVE

The posterior tibial nerve and its branches (the medial and lateral plantar nerves as well as the medial calcaneal nerve) can be entrapped within the tarsal tunnel, causing paresthesias and pain in the bottom of the foot (tarsal tunnel syndrome). The flexor tendons of the foot, in their own sheaths, (posterior tibial, flexor digitorum longus, and flexor hallucis longus) as well as the aforementioned neurovascular structures course behind the medial malleolus. The tarsal tunnel can be divided into upper (tibio-talar) and lower (talocalcaneal) tunnels.[12,13] The upper component is bordered by the deep fascia and the tibia and talus and contains the posterior tibial neurovascular structures. The lower portion of the tibial tunnel is bordered by the flexor retinaculum. In the imaging literature, the bony landmark of the sustentaculum talus has been used as a determination for this division of upper and lower tarsal tunnels.[4] However, in the surgical literature, the superior border of the abductor hallucis muscle is used. The tibial nerve divides into the medial and lateral plantar nerve deep to the flexor retinac-ulum 93% of the time but does occur proximally in the upper tunnel in 7%.[14] In the lower tarsal tunnel, the medial, lateral, and calcaneal nerves are separated by fibrous septae into distinct tunnels.[15,16]

A specific cause for tarsal tunnel syndrome can only be identified in 60% to 80% of patients.[17] The specific causes that can be prospectively identified with imaging include ganglion cysts or other masses, tenosynovitis of the flexor tendons, calcaneal fracture deformities, venous varicosities, and accessory muscles (**Figs. 4 and 5**).[5] One of the most common causes of tarsal tunnel syndrome, traction neuritis and perineural fibrosis, can be more difficult to ascertain with imaging. Evaluation of MRI for strandy areas of decreased T1 signal in the perineural fat with greater than 180 degrees contact with the adjacent nerve or areas of increased perineural acoustic impedance

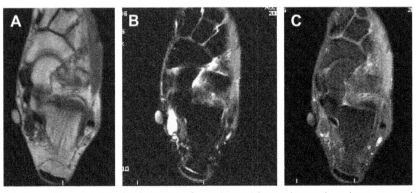

**Fig. 4.** Magnetic resonance (MR) images of a patient with tarsal tunnel syndrome secondary to a ganglion cyst in the lower tarsal tunnel. (*A*) Axial T1-weighted image shows a small oval mass within the tarsal tunnel at the level of the sustentaculum tali, with mass effect on the neurovascular structures posteriorly. (*B*) Axial T2-weighted image shows that the mass has homogeneously increased T2 signal. (*C*) Axial T1-weighted image with fat suppression after the administration of gadolinium contrast shows only faint peripheral wall enhancement, consistent with a cyst.

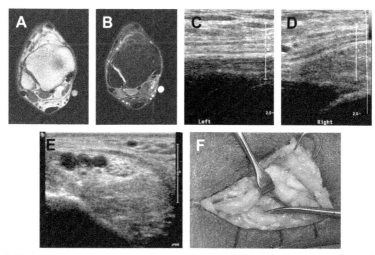

**Fig. 5.** Patient with tarsal tunnel syndrome secondary to a lipoma in the upper tarsal tunnel. (A) Axial T1-weighted MR image shows a subtle mass with T1 signal similar to subcutaneous fat immediately posterior to the tibial nerve. (B) Axial T2-weighted image with fat suppression shows that the mass has no increased T2 signal. (C) Longitudinal US of the normal tibial nerve in the contralateral side. (D) Longitudinal US shows the tibial nerve in the symptomatic side displaced anteriorly by the mass. (E) Transverse US image shows the posterior tibial artery, veins, and the enlarged nerve under the fascia being displaced by the posterior mass. (F) Surgical probe showing the relationship of the lipoma to the retracted neurovascular structures. (*Courtesy of* Dr John S. Gould, MD, Birmingham, AL.)

with decreased echogenicity on US is more subtle, but these can be diagnosed, when present, if careful attention is paid to technique.

Although imaging signs of direct tibial nerve dysfunction (increased T2 signal or enhancement with gadolinium contrast on MRI, or altered fascicle morphology and increased nerve size on US and MRI) can sometimes be found, it is more likely that the posterior tibial nerve will appear normal on imaging when no specific focal masses are present.[7,18]

Imaging of failed tarsal tunnel surgery can reveal possible incomplete retinacular release or postoperative scar, and may allow for improved preoperative mapping of the location of entrapment.[19,20]

## INFERIOR CALCANEAL NERVE

The inferior calcaneal nerve (first branch of the lateral plantar, or Baxter's nerve) originates from the lateral plantar nerve and initially travels deep to the abductor hallucis muscle. It then courses laterally, making a 90-degree turn at the inferior border of the abductor hallucis muscle to proceed in a horizontal direction between the quadratus plantus and the flexor digitorum brevis muscles. It passes anterior to the medial calcaneal tuberosity and innervates the adductor digiti minimi muscle.

Baxter's neuropathy is usually caused by a compression of the inferior calcaneal nerve.[4] It can occur at the point where the nerve turns horizontally between the quadratus plantae and flexor digitorum brevis, as described earlier, or from local pressure from an enthesophyte (bone spur) of the medial calcaneal tuberosity, as well as from severe plantar fasciitis in this location. Direct visualization of an enlarged inferior calcaneal nerve can be traced with a dedicated technique and high-resolution US.[7] With

MRI, recent publications have suggested a secondary finding that may suggest this diagnosis is diffuse muscle edema or fatty atrophy of the adductor digiti minimi from chronic denervation.[21,22] However, more recently, this finding has been found in 4% to 11% of normal volunteers without foot pain so the clinical relevance of fatty atrophy of the adductor digiti minimi muscle is uncertain.[23]

## DIGITAL NERVES

The medial plantar nerve proceeds distally under the medial aspect of the plantar foot, innervating the abductor hallucis, flexor hallucis brevis, and flexor digitorum brevis muscles, until it trifurcates into the intermetatarsal nerves of the medial 3 intermetatarsal spaces and terminates as the proper digital nerves. The medial plantar nerve can become entrapped at its location between the knot of Henry (the intersection of the flexor hallucis longus and flexor digitorum longus tendons) and the abductor hallucis muscle. The lateral plantar nerve bifurcates into a deep motor branch that innervates the interossei and lumbrical muscles and a superficial branch that terminates as the intermetatarsal nerve of the fourth intermetatarsal space.

Chronic repetitive trauma and impingement of the digital nerves leads to perineural fibrosis and the development of the Morton neuroma. This condition is most prevalent in women and has been attributed to footwear with high heels and a small toebox. The most common locations are the third and second intermetatarsal spaces. Both MRI and US can be used successfully in diagnosing Morton neuroma with sensitivities of 85% to 98% and specificities of 87% to 100%.[24]

MRI of the forefoot is performed with the patient prone to improve visualization of Morton neuroma. The intermetatarsal mass has typically decreased signal on T1 and T2-weighted images, although, if there is an adjacent intermetatarsal bursa, it may have increased T2 signal. It may also enhance after contrast administration (**Fig. 6**).[25]

On US, neuromas are identified as fusiform, noncompressible, hypoechoic masses displacing the expected hyperechoic fat within the intermetatarsal spaces (**Fig. 7**). They are typically seen immediately adjacent to the digital artery when using Doppler interrogation, but may not have an intralesional Doppler signal. Performing a sonographic Mulder test (squeezing the metatarsal bones together and visualizing the neuroma popping up plantarly) can improve the sensitivity.[26] Sometimes intermetatarsal

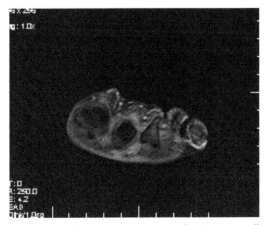

**Fig. 6.** Coronal T1 fat-suppressed, postcontrast image showing a small enhancing Morton neuroma in the second intermetatarsal space.

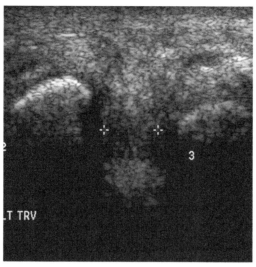

**Fig. 7.** Transverse US image of the second intermetatarsal space showing a hypoechoic mass (between the caliper markings) consistent with a Morton neuroma.

bursae can appear similar to neuromas and they can occur in association with underlying neuromas. To distinguish them from neuromas, compression with overlying transducer pressure is helpful.

US can also be used to direct therapeutic injections of local anesthetics and corticosteroids into the neuromas (**Fig. 8**). Injection of local anesthetic and corticosteroid into the neuroma may improve duration of short-term pain relief when compared with non–imaging-guided injections into the symptomatic webspace.[27,28] Injections of

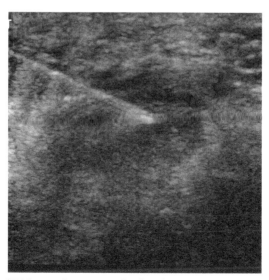

**Fig. 8.** Longitudinal US image shows a needle placed using direct sonographic guidance into a hypoechoic oval Morton neuroma in the second intermetatarsal space before injecting 20% alcohol as an ablating agent.

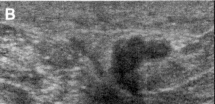

**Fig. 9.** Amputation neuroma at the site of scarring from prior sural neurectomy. (*A*) Longitudinal US images show the hypoechoic nerve ending in a fusiform oval mass near the prior surgical margin. (*B*) Transverse US image shows a large hypoechoic mass that proved to be amputation neuroma retracted into a surgical scar.

absolute ethyl alcohol into the neuroma can be performed via a dorsal approach. Care is taken to inject only into the Morton neuroma to avoid injury to the adjacent neurovascular structures. This procedure may need to be repeated up to 4 times, but a recent series has shown greater than 90% partial or complete relief of symptoms and decrease in size of the neuromas with this percutaneous treatment option. Postprocedure US shows a decrease in the size and an increase in the echogenicity of these masses.[29]

## SURAL NERVE

The sural nerve is a purely sensory nerve located in the subcutaneous fat along the lateral Achilles tendon, then coursing inferiorly below the lateral malleolus and the peroneal tendons and bifurcating into its terminal branches at the level of the fifth metatarsal base. Sural neuropathy may thus be secondary to tendinopathy of the adjacent Achilles and peroneal tendons or in the setting of prior trauma, the sequela of prior fractures involving the lateral malleolus of the ankle or foot bones such as the cuboid or base of the fifth metatarsal base.[4]

The lesser saphenous vein is adjacent to the sural nerve and allows accurate sonographic localization of this small nerve on its course down the calf near the Achilles tendon.[7] The sonographic findings of entrapment are previously described (focal enlargement before the site of entrapment and focal narrowing at site of entrapment from adjacent scarring or other extrinsic causes) (**Fig. 9**). MRI is less useful in directly

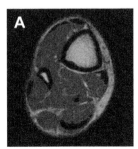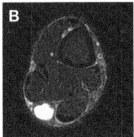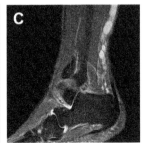

**Fig. 10.** Cystic mass with secondary sural nerve compression (*A*) Axial T1-weighted image shows the sural nerve displaced anteriorly by a low T1 mass. (*B*) Axial T2-weighted image shows that the mass has markedly increased T2 signal and a thin wall. (*C*) Sagittal T2 image shows a multilobulated mass with increased T2 signal at the expected location of the sural nerve. (*Courtesy of* Dr Brian Howard, Charlotte, NC.)

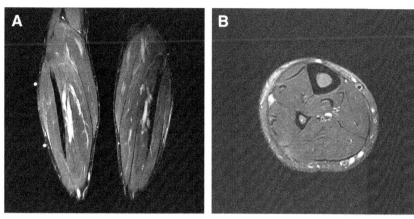

**Fig. 11.** A 26-year old runner with prior fasciotomies for chronic compression syndrome now with lateral calf, ankle and foot numbness. (*A*) Coronal T2-weighted image showing the fascial defect and strandy decreased signal in the subcutaneous fat at the site of the superficial peroneal nerve exiting the fascia, suggesting perineural fibrosis. (*B*) Axial T2-weighted image at the same level showing increased signal within the superficial peroneal nerve before exiting into the subcutaneous tissues of the anterolateral foreleg. (*Courtesy of* Dr Kenneth Wolfson, Charlotte, NC.)

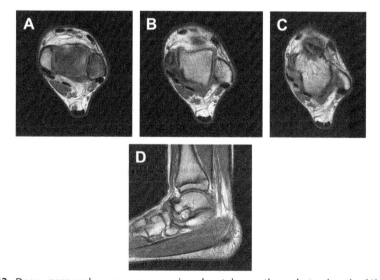

**Fig. 12.** Deep peroneal nerve compression by talar enthesophyte (spur). (*A*) Axial T1-weighted image just proximal to the talar enthesophyte. Note slightly enlarged neurovascular structure under the extensor retinaculum. (*B*) Axial T1-weighted image 3 mm distal to (*A*) showing capsular distension and enthesophyte encroaching the deep peroneal nerve. (*C*) Axial T1-weighted image 5.5 mm distal to (*B*) shows displacement of the nerve by the talar enthesophyte. (*D*) Sagittal T1-weighted image shows extent of enthesophyte and dorsal capsular distension encroaching on the deep peroneal nerve.

visualizing the sural nerve entrapment, given the small size of this nerve and its lack of motor function to allow for assessment of MRI denervation changes as previously described. However, MRI may be helpful in assessing the degree of tendinopathy or other underlying cause (**Fig. 10**).

## SUPERFICIAL AND DEEP PERONEAL NERVES

The common peroneal nerve branches into the superficial and deep peroneal nerves. The superficial peroneal nerve can be identified with US as it pierces the muscular fascia between the lateral and anterior muscle compartments approximately 12.5 cm above the lateral malleolus in most individuals.[30] This is a site of potential stretch injury, entrapment, and tethering, and imaging evaluation with MRI for adjacent muscle hernias, fascial inflammation, or thickening may be helpful in this area (**Fig. 11**). If the nerve pierces the deep fascia more distally, it may have a limited ability to resist a stretching injury and thus could be a predisposing factor for injury.[7]

After exiting the fascia, the superficial peroneal nerve then courses through the anterolateral subcutaneous tissues of the calf. It provides sensation to most of the dorsal surface of the foot via its 2 main branches (the intermediate and medial dorsal cutaneous nerves), sparing the first web space, which is innervated by the deep peroneal nerve. Injury to the distal nerve can occur from ankle trauma or arthroscopy.[30]

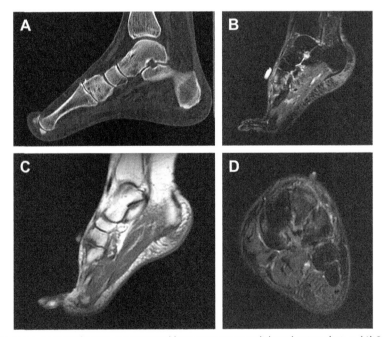

**Fig. 13.** Deep peroneal nerve compressed by tarsometatarsal dorsal osteophytes. (*A*) Sagittal images reformatted with computed tomography showing degenerative joint disease (DJD) in the great toe tarsometatarsal joint with dorsal osteophytes. (*B*) Sagittal T2-weighted image in a different patient shows DJD of the tarsometatarsal joint and edema in the dorsal soft tissues. (*C*) Sagittal T1-weighted image at the same location as (*B*) shows the DJD of the tarsometatarsal joint with subchondral sclerosis and dorsal osteophytes. (*D*) Coronal T2-weighted image of the same patient as (*B*) and (*C*) shows that the deep peroneal nerve is enlarged and has increased signal in this location.

Because the superficial peroneal nerve does not have an accompanying vascular structure, it can be difficult to localize with MRI or US without a good appreciation of its expected anatomic course.

The deep peroneal nerve courses within the anterior compartment of the calf, adjacent to the interosseous membrane and the anterior tibial vessels. It can be visualized most reliably in this deep location with MRI, but MRI is poor in its distal identification because of its small size and its close apposition to the dorsal surfaces of the foot bones.

Using US, the nerve can be well seen as it becomes more superficial under the extensor retinaculum between the extensor hallucis longus and extensor digitorum longus, just lateral to the dorsalis pedis artery. The deep peroneal nerve can be compressed at the inferior extensor retinaculum where the extensor hallucis longus tendon crosses over it (**Fig. 12**). The nerve then divides into a sensory branch for the first web space, as mentioned previously, and a motor branch to the extensor digitorum brevis muscle. The sensory branch of the deep peroneal nerve courses over the dorsum of the foot, so trauma in this area from tight shoewear, or repetitive blows as is seen with soccer players, can cause chronic injury.[7] It can also be entrapped between the extensor hallucis brevis tendon and the first and second tarsometatarsal joints, especially if there are dorsal osteophytes in the tarsometatarsal joints, secondary to underlying degenerative joint disease (**Fig. 13**).[31]

## REFERENCES

1. Gold GE, Suh B, Sawyer-Glover A, et al. Musculoskeletal MRI at 3.0 T: initial clinical experience. AJR Am J Roentgenol 2004;183(5):1479–86.
2. Aagard BD, Lazar DA, Lankerovich L, et al. High resolution magnetic resonance imaging is a non-invasive method of observing injury and recovery in the peripheral nervous system. Neurosurgery 2003;53(1):199–203.
3. Allen JM, Greer BJ, Sorge DG, et al. MR imaging of neuropathies of the leg, ankle, and foot. Magn Reson Imaging Clin N Am 2008;16(1):117–31, vii.
4. Delfaut EM, Demondion X, Bieganski A, et al. Imaging of foot and ankle nerve entrapment syndromes: from well-demonstrated to unfamiliar sites. Radiographics 2003;23(3):613–23.
5. Donovan A, Rosenberg ZS, Cavalcanti CF. MR imaging of entrapment neuropathies of the lower extremity. Part 2. The knee, leg, ankle, and foot. Radiographics 2010;30(4):1001–19.
6. McMahon CJ, Wu JS, Eisenberg RL. Muscle edema. AJR Am J Roentgenol 2010; 194:W284–92.
7. Martinoli C, Court Payon M, Michaud J, et al. Imaging of neuropathies about the ankle and foot. Semin Musculoskelet Radiol 2010;14(3):344–56.
8. Martinoli C, Bianchi S, Derchi LE. Tendon and nerve sonography. Radiol Clin North Am 1999;37(4):691–711.
9. Abrahams MS, Aziz MF, Fu RF, et al. Ultrasound guidance compared with electrical neurostimulation for peripheral nerve block: a systematic review and meta-analysis of randomized controlled trials. Br J Anaesth 2009;102(3):408–17.
10. Redborg KE, Antonakakis JG, Beach ML, et al. Ultrasound improves the success rate of a tibial nerve block at the ankle. Reg Anesth Pain Med 2009; 34(3):256–60.
11. Redborg KE, Sites BD, Chinn CD, et al. Ultrasound improves the success rate of a sural nerve block at the ankle. Reg Anesth Pain Med 2009;34(1):24–8.
12. Zeiss J, Fenton P, Ebraheim N, et al. Normal magnetic resonance anatomy of the tarsal tunnel. Foot Ankle 1990;10(4):214–8.

13. Erickson SJ, Quinn SF, Kneeland JB, et al. MR imaging of the tarsal tunnel and related spaces: normal and abnormal findings with anatomic correlation. AJR Am J Roentgenol 1990;155(2):323–8.
14. Havel PE, Ebraheim NA, Clark SE, et al. Tibial nerve branching in the tarsal tunnel. Foot Ankle 1988;9(3):117–9.
15. Dellon AL. The four medial ankle tunnels: a critical review of perceptions of tarsal tunnel syndrome and neuropathy. Neurosurg Clin N Am 2008;19(4):629–48.
16. Franson J, Baravarian B. Tarsal tunnel syndrome: a compression neuropathy involving four distinct tunnels. Clin Podiatr Med Surg 2006;23(3):597–609.
17. Lau JT, Daniels TR. Tarsal tunnel syndrome: a review of the literature. Foot Ankle Int 1999;20(3):201–9.
18. Nagaoka M, Matsuzaki H. Ultrasonography in tarsal tunnel syndrome. J Ultrasound Med 2005;24(8):1035–40.
19. Zeiss J, Fenton P, Ebraheim N, et al. Magnetic resonance imaging for ineffectual tarsal tunnel surgical treatment. Clin Orthop Relat Res 1991;264:264–6.
20. Raikin SM, Minnich JM. Failed tarsal tunnel syndrome surgery. Foot Ankle Clin 2003;8(1):159–74.
21. Recht MP, Grooff P, Ilaslan H, et al. Selective atrophy of the abductor digiti quinti: an MRI study. AJR Am J Roentgenol 2007;189:W123–7.
22. Chundru U, Liebeskind A, Seidelmann F, et al. Plantar fasciitis and calcaneal spur formation are associated with abductor digiti minimi atrophy on MRI of the foot. Skeletal Radiol 2008;37(6):505–10.
23. Schmid DT, Hodler J, Mengiardi B, et al. Fatty muscle atrophy: prevalence in the hindfoot muscles on MR images of asymptomatic volunteers and patients with foot pain. Radiology 2009;253(1):160–6.
24. Zanetti M, Strehle JK, Kundert HP, et al. Morton neuroma: effect of MR imaging findings on diagnostic thinking and therapeutic decisions. Radiology 1999;213(2):583–8.
25. Terk MR, Kwong PK, Suthar M, et al. Morton neuroma: evaluation with MR imaging performed with contrast enhancement and fat suppression. Radiology 1993;189:239–41.
26. Torriani M, Kattapuram SV. Technical innovation: dynamic sonography of the forefoot. The sonographic Mulder sign. AJR Am J Roentgenol 2003;180:1121–3.
27. Markovic M, Crichton K, Read JW, et al. Effectiveness of ultrasound-guided corticosteroid injection in the treatment of Morton's neuroma. Foot Ankle Int 2008;29(5):483–7.
28. Sofka CM, Adler RS, Ciavarra GA, et al. Ultrasound-guided interdigital neuroma injections: short-term clinical outcomes after a single percutaneous injection–preliminary results. HSS J 2007;3(1):44–9.
29. Hughes RJ, Ali K, Jones H, et al. Treatment of Morton's neuroma with alcohol injection under sonographic guidance: follow-up of 101 cases. AJR Am J Roentgenol 2007;188(6):1535–9.
30. Canella C, Demondion X, Guillin R, et al. Anatomic study of the superficial peroneal nerve using sonography. AJR Am J Roentgenol 2009;193:174–9.
31. Parker RG. Dorsal foot pain due to compression of the deep peroneal nerve by exostosis of the metatarsocuneiform joint. J Am Podiatr Med Assoc 2005;95(5):455–8.

# Electrodiagnostic Evaluation of Lower Extremity Neurogenic Problems

Paige C. Roy, MD

**KEYWORDS**

- Electrodiagnosis • Electromyography
- Nerve conduction studies • Lower extremity • Foot • Ankle

Electrodiagnosis is a powerful tool in the evaluation of lower extremity disorders that stem from the peripheral nervous system. Electrodiagnostic testing can help differentiate neurogenic versus non-neurogenic causes of complaints such as pain, weakness, and paresthesias. It can assist practitioners in pinpointing the anatomic location and revealing the underlying pathology in peripheral nerve lesions. This article will focus on the electrodiagnostic evaluation of neurogenic processes that present as foot and ankle symptoms.

## ELECTRODIAGNOSIS BASICS

To discuss this subject in detail, the basics components of electrodiagnosis (EDx) must be understood. Typically the electrodiagnostic medicine consultation involves a focused history and physical examination performed by a qualified electromyographer, development of a differential diagnosis, and two test components: nerve conduction studies (NCS) and electromyography (EMG). The term EMG is frequently used to refer to both components of the test, but it is important to recognize the individual components' value and how they differ from and complement each other.

### NCS

NCS involve the application of a small controlled electrical stimulus to a peripheral nerve with recording of the subsequent response. Responses are most commonly recorded with surface electrodes on the patient's skin. Both sensory nerves and motor nerves can be evaluated with NCS. The recorded sensory nerve action potential is frequently labeled as a SNAP. The recorded motor nerve action potential is frequently

The author has nothing to disclose.

Department of Physical Medicine and Rehabilitation, The University of Alabama at Birmingham, 1201 11th Avenue South, Suite 100, Birmingham, AL 35205, USA

E-mail address: pcroy@uab.edu

labeled as a CMAP (compound motor action potential). A mixed nerve action potential resulting from a combined sensory and motor nerve response can also be recorded.

Some of the important parameters analyzed in NCS include the conduction velocity, latency, and amplitude of each response. The latency is a measure of time and is determined by the conduction velocity of the nerve fibers. Latency is typically determined from the time the stimulus occurs to the time the evoked potential appears (measured either at the onset or peak of the recorded potential).

When recording a SNAP, the amplitude is indicative of the total number of sensory axons that depolarize in the sensory nerve being tested. Decreased SNAP amplitudes suggest a peripheral nerve disorder, specifically distal to the dorsal root ganglion (DRG). Such lesions are often labeled postganglionic. The DRG contains the sensory nerve cell bodies and is typically located in the intervertebral foramen. This has important anatomic consideration when interpreting NCS results. Lesions that are proximal to the DRG or preganglionic, such a radiculopathies, generally show preservation of the SNAP responses.[1] However, in postganglionic processes, such as plexopathies or more distal peripheral nerve lesions, the SNAPs recorded often reflect damage to the sensory nerve axons.

With a CMAP, the amplitude is a reflection of the number of muscle fibers activated with the stimulus. CMAP amplitudes can be decreased by motor nerve axon loss to the muscle over which the response is recorded.[1] The CMAP amplitude can also be affected by muscle atrophy, muscle fiber damage, or neuromuscular transmission defects. It is important to specify which muscle or region the CMAP is being recorded from to properly interpret the findings. For example, a peroneal motor NCS recorded over the tibialis anterior (TA) may be normal, while the same peroneal motor nerve conduction recorded over the extensor digitorum brevis (EDB) may reflect an abnormality.

The results of a patient's NCS are typically compared with known normal values for each nerve evaluated. In addition, NCS of an individual nerve should be compared with other nerves tested within the patient's affected limb. In some cases, it may be necessary to study the analogous contralateral nerve to establish the existence of an abnormality. Because of the possible variation in side-to-side comparison, a decrease in amplitude of 50% is often used to indicate the presence of pathology.

### Electromyography

EMG involves a disposable needle electrode that is placed in various muscles to evaluate their bioelectrical activity. The clinical question, history and physical examination, and abnormalities found as the study progresses determine the muscles that are examined. Detailed anatomic knowledge is necessary to accurately perform the EMG examination and make thoughtful conclusions. Pathology involving the peripheral nerve, neuromuscular junction, or muscle may be seen with EMG. Typically EMG includes evaluation of insertional activity, abnormal spontaneous activity, and motor unit action potentials.

Insertional activity (IA) is observed when the needle is being moved through the muscle in small increments. A muscle should be relatively electrically silent when the needle and muscle are at rest. IA is recorded when the needle is moved and a small burst of potentials is evoked by local muscle fiber depolarization. IA can be labeled as normal, increased (typical in denervation processes or muscle fiber damage), or decreased (typical with muscle atrophy).

The abnormal spontaneous activity seen in EMG is most frequently noted as the presence of fibrillations (Fibs) or positive sharp waves (PSWs). Fibs and PSWs result from the abnormal spontaneous firing of a single muscle fiber. These abnormal potentials may be present in denervation of a muscle fiber (neurogenic processes) or damage to a muscle fiber (myopathic processes or trauma).

Motor unit action potential (MUAP) analysis occurs when the patient is asked to contract the muscle in which the needle is placed. The resulting MUAPs are then evaluated based upon their waveform morphology (amplitude, duration, and complexity/phases) and recruitment (the orderly pattern in which normal motor units activate). MUAP abnormalities occur in both neurogenic and myopathic processes but have distinct differences that enable differentiation. Further details of MUAP analysis are beyond the scope of this article but can be found in other sources.

The anatomic pattern of EMG abnormalities seen in EDx helps pinpoint the particular peripheral nerve or group of peripheral nerves involved. EMG can be helpful in analyzing nerve segments that are not easily measured by surface electrodes in NCS (ie, proximal limb muscles/nerves). EMG can also provide definitive evidence of axon loss by the presence of abnormal spontaneous activity. It can also be used to measure the degree of remaining evocable motor units in an injured nerve.

## PERIPHERAL NERVE ASSESSMENT

It is important to note that EDx evaluates the integrity of the peripheral nervous system (PNS) and is not diagnostic in central nervous system disorders. When a PNS disorder is present, EDx can be used to characterize the type of pathology (myopathic vs neuropathic, axon loss vs demyelination), assess the severity and chronicity of the pathology, and localize the anatomic site of the abnormalities.

Peripheral nerve disorders can result from axonal loss or demyelinative lesions or can be a combination of both. When axonal damage occurs at a focal point in the nerve, the distal portion of the nerve begins to undergo Wallerian degeneration. Axon damage is frequently reflected in the amplitude of the SNAP and CMAP and the presence of abnormal spontaneous activity on EMG. With complete axonal disruption, the CMAP may be preserved for 7 days while the SNAP may take 10 days to disappear. EMG findings of denervation (Fibs and PSW) may take greater than 3 weeks to develop and are dependent upon how far the lesion site is away from the muscle being tested.[1]

Thus the timing of EDx testing is important to consider. Following a known nerve insult, it is often recommended one wait at least 3 weeks before pursuing EDx testing. Before this time period limited information can be obtained, and the results may not accurately reflect the precise anatomic location or degree of abnormality present.

Other peripheral nerve lesions may result in focal demyelination. This frequently results in slowing of conduction and may be seen on NCS as decreased conduction velocity or delayed distal latency of the affected nerve. Demyelination may also result in blockade of some or all of the nerve impulses across the lesion. This is frequently termed conduction block. If it is a purely demyelinative lesion that does not affect the underlying axons, Wallerian degeneration does not occur. Thus stimulation distal to the lesion site will produce normal SNAP and CMAP responses. When stimulation occurs proximal to the lesion, however, the neural impulses may be blocked and result in decreased amplitudes of the CMAP or SNAP.[1] The needle EMG examination in purely demyelinative processes may be normal or show only mild decreased motor unit recruitment. In such cases, abnormal spontaneous activity would not be expected to be present on EMG.

When evaluating the health of peripheral nerves, especially in traumatic nerve injury, it is important to remember two additional points. The existence of voluntary motor units on EMG testing indicates some degree of axon continuity. If no motor units are evocable on attempted activation of the muscle, this can indicate lack of axon continuity or complete conduction block.

### History and Physical Examination

One of the most important steps in the initial evaluation of foot and ankle complaints by an electromyographer is eliciting an appropriately detailed but focused history of the complaints. A patient's history of pain, weakness, or paresthesias and their specific anatomic distribution should be explored. It is important to elicit from the patient whether the symptoms were insidious or sudden-onset, whether they are intermittent or continuous, and any relative progression. Certainly, the differential diagnosis for a patient who presents with complaints of sudden-onset numbness in a focal nerve distribution after a fall would likely vary from a patient with gradual-onset progressive numbness in both feet. The past medical history, especially known endocrine, rheumatologic, neurologic, and orthopedic disorders should be obtained. Other important history includes any related trauma, temporally related illness, hospitalization, surgery, or interventional procedure.

The physical examination is also a key piece in the electrodiagnostic consultation. A sensory and motor examination should be performed with consideration of whether the abnormalities seen reflect a peripheral nerve, dermatomal, or myotomal distribution. Notation of muscle atrophy or other asymmetry should be made. Provocative testing such as a Tinel sign over a peripheral nerve or a positive straight leg raise test may help focus the differential further. The history and physical examination details help an electromyographer construct an appropriate EDx testing plan and ultimately provide a clinically relevant interpretation.

Electrodiagnostic testing can help delineate the precise anatomic location of the peripheral nerve lesion and assess the degree of nerve damage. It can also assist with therapeutic decision making by pinpointing an area to image or surgically intervene. The presence of overlapping peripheral neurologic processes may also be detected, which may affect treatment and prognosis.

The remaining portion of this article will be dedicated to discussing the specific pathologic PNS processes that might present with foot and ankle complaints and how EDx can help in meaningful clinical differentiation of these disorders. Focal entrapment neuropathies, lumbosacral radiculopathies and plexopathies, and peripheral polyneuropathies will be discussed.

## FOCAL ENTRAPMENT NEUROPATHIES

Focal entrapment neuropathies may result from a slowly compressive lesion or traumatic damage to a nerve. This can result in demyelination or axonal loss and may affect sensory or motor nerves depending on the location of the lesion. Sensory and motor NCS should be performed in the affected region. In focal peripheral neuropathies, the sensory fibers are frequently affected first and more severely. This often results in SNAP abnormalities before changes in the CMAP are seen. As the lesion progresses, CMAP changes may become more evident.

EMG is a particularly useful tool for determining the anatomic distribution of abnormalities. The needle can be used to access muscles that are difficult to assess with NCS and surface electrodes. Therefore EMG is extremely helpful in localizing processes to a specific peripheral nerve, plexus, or root pattern. The electromyographer interprets the data gained from both NCS and EMG to form a relevant clinical diagnosis.

## Common Peroneal Nerve

Following its departure from the peroneal division of the sciatic nerve in the region of the knee, the common peroneal nerve (CPN) descends around the fibular head and splits into its superficial and deep branches. Trauma (eg, fracture or laceration) can cause injury anywhere along its anatomic course. However, the most frequent peroneal neuropathy seen is a common peroneal neuropathy at the fibular head. This may occur from external compression or stretch injury as the result of surgical or bed positioning, prolonged squatting or leg crossing, proximal fibular fractures, knee arthroscopy or arthroplasty,[2] and severe ankle sprains. It is the most common lower limb peripheral nerve injury after polytrauma, especially motor vehicle accidents.[3]

Common peroneal neuropathies at the fibular head may result in weakness of the toe and ankle dorsiflexors and foot evertors. A Tinel sign may be present over the CPN at the fibular head. Sensory loss and subjective paresthesias can vary and depend upon the degree of nerve damage. In severe injuries, sensation should be diminished in the anteriolateral distal leg and dorsal foot including the first web space. If the sensory or motor abnormalities seen on physical examination are more diffuse, a more proximal lesion should be suspected.

Electrodiagnostic studies should include superficial peroneal sensory NCS and common peroneal motor NCS recorded at EDB. The common peroneal motor NCS should include stimulation at the ankle, below the fibular head, and above the fibular head at the level of the knee. Classically, a common peroneal neuropathy at the fibular head should reflect abnormalities in the superficial peroneal SNAP. The CMAP may show decreased conduction velocity or conduction block across the fibular head. Of note, in severe cases, the EDB is often profoundly affected and limits interpretation of the motor NCS. If the CMAP recording at the EDB shows a severely diminished response, then recording at the TA may be required to demonstrate a focal area of decreased conduction across the fibular head.[4] Comparison ipsilateral sural sensory and tibial motor NCS also should be performed. If the sural or tibial NCS are abnormal, then a search for a more proximal lesion or a more diffuse process must occur.

A common peroneal neuropathy at the fibular head should show EMG changes in both the superficial and deep peroneal supplied muscles. Of note, frequently muscles supplied by the superficial peroneal branch (ie, peroneus longus) are less affected than those supplied by the deep branch (ie, EDB, TA). These muscles should be evaluated along with comparison tibial, sciatic, and more proximal supplied L4, L5, S1 muscles. It is also important to examine the short head of the biceps femoris with EMG. An abnormality in this muscle would suggest that the nerve lesion is actually proximal to the knee, either in the peroneal division of the sciatic nerve, or more proximal at the sciatic nerve, plexus, or root level.

Of note, a frequent mimicker of a common peroneal neuropathy with resultant foot drop is a L5 radiculopathy. To evaluate for this possibility, additional muscles should be tested. EMG of the lumbosacral paraspinals, posterior tibialis, tensor fascia lata, or gluteus medius may help with further localization.[1] This is especially true in cases that do not demonstrate the classic NCS findings.

## Deep Peroneal Nerve

Distal to the fibular head, the CPN splits to give rise to the deep and superficial peroneal nerves. The deep peroneal nerve (DPN) descends to innervate the muscles of the anterior compartment of the leg and sensation to the first web space. The DPN can become entrapped at the anterior ankle under the inferior extensor retinaculum. This is sometimes referred to as anterior tarsal tunnel syndrome, and it can affect the sensory and/or motor branches of the DPN. The motor branch supplies the EDB muscle. If the sensory branch is affected, patients typically complain of paresthesias within the first web space. If the motor branch is affected, the patient may complain of pain across the dorsal foot and ankle. Nocturnal exacerbation of these symptoms may occur as well. Weakness of the EDB is often not perceived by patients, but if severe, atrophy of the EDB may be appreciated. A Tinel sign may be present over the DPN at the anterior ankle.

This disorder may occur after trauma, especially when a heavy item is dropped onto the surface, compressing the DPN. Excessively tight or rigid footwear has also been proposed as a mechanism of injury. Ankle plantar flexion with simultaneous dorsiflexion of the toes, as seen in high-heeled shoe wear, is also thought to stress the DPN at the ankle.[5,6]

Electrophysiologic evaluation should include the deep peroneal sensory NCS. However, it should be noted that this SNAP is particularly small and may be technically challenging to record even in normal individuals. Side-to-side comparison is recommended if possible. If the responses are absent bilaterally and the complaints are unilateral, extreme caution should be used in interpreting these electrical findings. The comparison ipsilateral superficial peroneal and sural sensory NCS should be performed and should be normal in anterior tarsal tunnel syndrome (**Fig. 1, Table 1**).

The DPN should be stimulated at the ankle and the CMAP recorded at the EDB. Contralateral comparison of this study can further assist with documentation of the focal lesion and the degree of axon loss. The ipsilateral tibial motor NCS recorded at the abductor hallucis (AH) is also helpful to further exclude a more diffuse process such as a peripheral polyneuropathy.[7] The peroneal CMAP recording should also include stimulation below and above the fibular head to exclude the more frequently seen common peroneal neuropathy at the fibular head. A unilateral prolongation of the distal latency, or decreased amplitude of the CMAP recorded at the EDB, with preservation of proximal conduction, is suggestive of a focal deep peroneal lesion.[8]

However, in patients without the classic symptomatology, isolated decreased CMAP amplitude recorded at the EDB should be interpreted with caution. Local foot trauma or surgical history in this area may affect NCS/EMG results. Congenitally absent EDB muscles have been also been described.[9,10]

In a pure focal entrapment of the DPN at the ankle, EMG changes are classically isolated to the EDB. Evidence may include increased IA, abnormal spontaneous activity, or motor unit morphology, and recruitment changes may be seen in the affected foot's EDB. Electromyography of the contralateral EDB, ipsilateral tibial supplied intrinsic foot muscles, and more proximal peroneal and L5-S1 supplied muscles should be normal. Of note, typically the first dorsal interosseous pedis (DIP) is supplied by the lateral plantar branch of the tibial nerve. However, the DPN may also supply some motor branches to the medial interosseus muscles, especially the first DIP.[11,12] Therefore, EMG of other tibial supplied muscles in the foot (such as AH) may be more helpful in excluding tibial nerve involvement in the presence of a DPN neuropathy.

Of note, there is some controversy in the literature regarding the interpretation of EMG abnormalities in foot muscles. Some previous studies have described variable numbers of asymptomatic people as having prolonged IA without frank sustained abnormal spontaneous activity in the EDB and other intrinsic foot muscles.[11,13] Of note, these studies did not perform NCS on these asymptomatic people to evaluate for subclinical nerve dysfunction. The presence of these findings has been proposed to result from wear and tear of the foot.[11,13] It is this author's experience and opinion, as well as others,[11,14] that EMG evaluation of the foot is critical in the assessment of distal tibial and peroneal neuropathies. Sustained abnormal spontaneous activity and

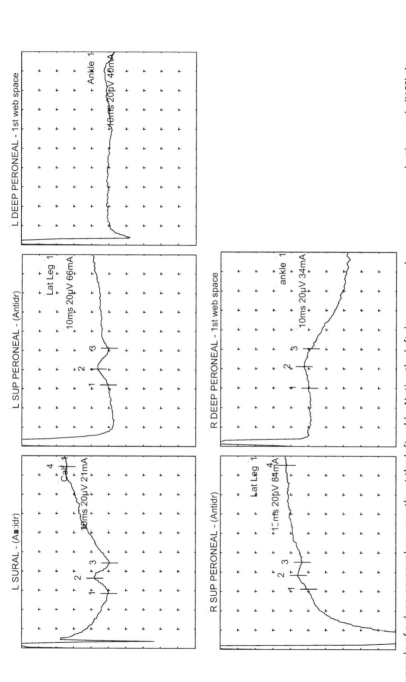

**Fig. 1.** Example of a deep peroneal neuropathy at the left ankle. Notice the left deep peroneal sensory nerve conduction study (NCS) shows no response, whereas the comparison right deep peroneal sensory nerve action potential (SNAP) is normal. The bilateral superficial peroneal SNAPs are normal and comparable to each other. Also, the ipsilateral left sural SNAP is normal. (Not shown: this patient also demonstrated decreased amplitude left peroneal compound motor action potential (CMAP) recorded at the extensor digitorum brevis (EDB) on side-to-side comparison. This motor NCS also showed normal conduction velocity throughout, without slowing across the fibular head. Electromyography (EMG) showed abnormalities limited only to the left EDB.)

**Table 1**
Sensory nerve conduction studies

| Nerve/Sites | Rec. Site | Onset Lat ms | Peak Lat ms | NP Amp μV | PP Amp μV | Segments | Distance cm | Velocity m/s | Area μVms |
|---|---|---|---|---|---|---|---|---|---|
| L Sural-(Antidr) | | | | | | | | | |
| Calf | Lat Mall | 2.85 | 3.65 | 16.0 | 17.1 | Calf-Lat Mall | 14 | 49.1 | 12.0 |
| L Sup Peroneal-(Antidr) | | | | | | | | | |
| Lat Leg | Ankle | 3.20 | 4.05 | 11.7 | 12.7 | Lat Leg-Ankle | 14 | 43.8 | 11.7 |
| L Deep Peroneal-1st Web Space | | | | | | | | | |
| Ankle | 1st web space | NR | NR | NR | NR | Ankle-1st web space | 14 | NR | NR |
| R Sup Peroneal-(Antidr) | | | | | | | | | |
| Lat Leg | Ankle | 3.10 | 3.85 | 11.0 | 4.5 | Lat Leg-Ankle | 14 | 45.2 | 6.3 |
| R Deep Peroneal-1st Web Space | | | | | | | | | |
| Ankle | 1st web space | 2.90 | 4.10 | 6.0 | 7.4 | Ankle-1st web space | 12 | 41.3 | 7.0 |

*Abbreviations:* Amp, amplitude; Antidr, antidromic; cm, centimeter; L, left; Lat, lateral; Mall, malleolus; ms, milliseconds; m/s, meters/second; NP, negative to peak; NR, no response; Onset Lat, onset latency; Peak Lat, peak latency; PP, peak to peak; R, right; Rec, recording; μV, microvolt.

MUAP abnormalities in an isolated nerve distribution in the foot that are consistent with the NCS findings, in this author's opinion, are strongly suspicious for a focal pathologic process. Combining an internally consistent EDx study with the relevant history and physical examination findings can also help strengthen diagnostic conclusions as previously discussed. Nevertheless, caution should be used when interpreting these electrodiagnostic findings, especially for less experienced practitioners.

### Superficial Peroneal Nerve

The superficial peroneal nerve (SPN) arises from the CPN and descends to innervate the peroneus longus and brevis muscles. The SPN then typically becomes a purely sensory nerve supplying sensation to the dorsal ankle and foot. The SPN can be traumatized anywhere along its anatomic course from lacerations or blunt trauma. A proximal SPN lesion may result in denervation in the previously mentioned muscles and changes in the superficial peroneal SNAP. More commonly however, the SPN can become entrapped above the ankle, where it pierces the deep fascia about 10 to 13 cm proximal to the lateral malleolus.[11,15] It may be injured with inversion ankle sprains, local trauma, or with muscle herniation through this fascial opening.[16] Injury of the SPN at this location can result in paresthesias and pain across the dorsal ankle and foot. Sensory examination classically demonstrates sparing the first web space and plantar foot. Muscle strength should also be preserved.

Electrophysiologic evaluation of a SPN lesion at the ankle most commonly shows decreased amplitude of the superficial peroneal SNAP when compared with the unaffected limb. The distal latency and conduction velocity are less commonly prolonged.[17] The peroneal motor NCS recorded at the EDB and the tibial motor NCS should be normal. EMG of all muscles tested, including the EDB, should be normal unless an accessory peroneal nerve is present as will be described.

Previous studies have estimated that approximately 28% of the population has an accessory DPN that branches off the SPN and courses around the lateral malleolus to supply a portion of the EDB.[18] This is considered an anatomic variant and in normal subjects has little consequence. However, it may serve as a source of confusion when performing EDx testing. Proof of its existence is relatively simple with routine NCS in normal individuals. However, in patients with peroneal neuropathies, the presence of an accessory DPN necessitates careful electrodiagnostic study and interpretation.[18]

### Sural Nerve

In the popliteal fossa, the sciatic nerve splits into the peroneal and tibial divisions becoming the peroneal and tibial nerves. The tibial nerve gives rise to the sural nerve (medial sural nerve) at the popliteal fossa. At the level of the mid-calf, this is joined by a communicating branch of the peroneal nerve (lateral sural nerve) to form the sural nerve proper. The sural nerve provides sensation to the lateral ankle and heel and the lateral edge of the foot.[1]

Isolated sural neuropathies are rare but can occur with local trauma, fibrotic bands, fractures, or ganglia.[19] Studies have shown it is the most common nerve injured in ankle arthroscopies followed by the SPN.[20] If injured, the patient may complain of paresthesias or pain in the distribution described previously. If deficits in sensation are found outside of the sural nerve territory, a more proximal lesion, such as a sciatic neuropathy, or a more diffuse neurogenic process, such as a peripheral polyneuropathy, should be considered. It is important to note that strength should also be normal. Any decreased strength in the leg or foot muscles should lead to suspicion of an alternative lesion location.

Electrodiagnostic evaluation of a focal sural neuropathy is relatively straightforward. Only the sural SNAP in the affected limb should show abnormalities.[1] Typically an ipsilateral superficial peroneal sensory NCS and a contralateral comparison sural sensory NCS should be performed to rule out the presence of a more diffuse disorder. It should be noted that the sural sensory NCS is thought to be one of the most sensitive NCS for detecting a peripheral polyneuropathy.[7] Therefore careful analysis is recommended to rule out this disorder. All motor NCS and EMG studies should be normal in the affected limb given the purely sensory nature of the sural nerve.

### Tibial Nerve

As the tibial nerve descends from the popliteal fossa it supplies the plantar flexors of the foot, the long toe flexors, posterior tibialis, and all intrinsic foot muscles of the foot except the EDB. It also branches to supply the sural nerve as described previously. At the ankle, the tibial nerve passes posterior to the medial malleolus and passes under the flexor retinaculum in the tarsal tunnel. In this region, the tibial nerve typically divides into four main branches to supply the majority of the intrinsic foot muscles and sensation to the plantar surface of the foot.

### Politeal fossa

Isolated tibial neuropathies in the region of popliteal fossa are relatively rare, but can result from Baker cysts, knee dislocation, or other focal trauma. If injured in this region, the patient may show weakness in the plantar flexors of the toes and foot, and sensory deficits in the sural distribution and the plantar surface of the foot. Patients may be able to walk on their toes but not their heels. There should be preservation of sensation and strength in the peroneal distribution. If the tibial nerve is damaged distal to the innervation of the gastrocnemius, the patient may demonstrate toe flexor weakness with relatively normal ankle plantar flexion. Sensation abnormalities should be limited to the plantar foot surface with sparing of the sural nerve distribution.

Electrodiagnostic evaluation of tibial neuropathies proximal to the ankle should include routine tibial and peroneal motor NCS of the affected limb. The tibial CMAP recorded at the AH may show decreased amplitude or conduction delay. Any peroneal CMAP abnormality should bring into question a more proximal process such as a sciatic neuropathy, plexopathy, or radiculopathy. The sural and superficial peroneal sensory NCS should also be performed. If the lesion is in the popliteal fossa, the sural SNAP should be affected. Again, contralateral comparison may be helpful in delineating this. If the lesion is distal in the mid-calf, then the sural SNAP is typically spared. The superficial peroneal SNAP should be normal.

As always, EMG abnormalities depend on the lesion location. The peroneal-supplied muscles and the more proximal sciatic and L5-S1 root-supplied muscles (gluteal and lumbosacral paraspinals muscles) should be normal in an isolated tibial neuropathy. EMG changes in the long toe flexors and the tibial supplied foot intrinsics, with relative sparing of the gastrocnemius muscles, would localize the lesion to the mid-calf. Abnormalities of the gastrocnemius muscles on EMG would localize the lesion to the area of the popliteal fossa or distal thigh.

### Foot and ankle

In the region of the tarsal tunnel, the tibial nerve divides into its four main branches: the medial and lateral plantar, and the medial and inferior calcaneal nerves. Previous studies have shown that in 93% to 95% of cases, the tibial nerve divides into the medial plantar nerve (MPN) and the lateral plantar nerve (LPN) within the tarsal tunnel. In the remainder of cases, this branching may occur above the flexor retinaculum.[21,22]

The MPN gives motor supply to the AH, first lumbrical, flexor digitorum brevis (FDB), and medial and lateral heads of the flexor hallucis brevis (FHB). The MPN provides sensation to the plantar first through third toes, medial half of the fourth toe, and medial sole of the foot.[11]

The LPN gives motor supply to a large portion of the intrinsic foot muscles, including all of the interrosseus muscles, second to fourth lumbricals, quadratus plantae (QP), flexor digitorum minimi brevis (FDMB), AH, and lateral head of the FHB. The LPN provides sensation to plantar fifth toe, lateral half of the fourth toe, and lateral sole of the foot.[11]

Branching of the medial calcaneal nerve (MCN) is highly variable and may occur within, distal, or proximal to the tarsal tunnel, and this may originate from the tibial nerve proper or the LPN.[21,22] The MCN is a purely sensory nerve and supplies sensation to the medial, posterior, and plantar heel.

The inferior calcaneal nerve (ICN) (also called Baxter's nerve) may branch from the tibial nerve proper. The ICN also may be the first branch of the lateral plantar nerve, and it is frequently labeled as such on anatomic diagrams.[21,22] After branching, the ICN eventually crosses anterior to the medial calcaneal tuberosity. The ICN does not provide cutaneous innervation to the foot. It may provide periosteal branches to the calcaneus and motor supply to the FDB or QP muscles. However, it always terminates in the abductor digiti quinti pedis (ADQP).[11]

Given the variable branching and complex nature of the tibial nerve anatomy in the tarsal tunnel region, detailed anatomic knowledge of the foot is required for electrodiagnostic evaluation. The etiologies for tarsal tunnel syndrome are too numerous to be listed here but include traumatic, compressive, biomechanical, and inflammatory disorders. The clinical and anatomic presentation of lesions of the tibial nerve branches can vary considerably. Therefore, it is this author's preference to avoid using the terminology tarsal tunnel syndrome, and instead label the individual nerve lesions by the branches they involve based upon the complete EDx consultation.

The clinical presentation of a distal tibial neuropathy in the tarsal tunnel region varies depending on the branches involved. It may include numbness, tingling, aching, burning, cramping, tightness, or other painful symptom in the distribution of the nerves affected. Classically, it is thought that prolonged ambulation or standing may exacerbate the symptoms. Nocturnal exacerbation is also frequently described. Often patients do not notice weakness or atrophy of the foot muscles unless it is severe.[11] However, careful clinical evaluation by the physician may reveal abnormalities in the bulk and strength of the foot muscles in more advanced cases. A Tinel sign may be positive over the involved nerve branch. Sensory changes in the distribution of the nerves involved may be elicited on testing. It should be noted that if the MCN branches above the flexor retinaculum, sensation to the heel may be spared even with fairly significant compression of the MPN and LPN in this region.

Electrophysiologic evaluation of the foot can be complex, technically challenging, and time consuming. Thoughtful performance and interpretation are critical in electrodiagnostic testing of the foot and should be performed by experienced electromyographers. Complete details of the EDx examination of the foot are beyond the scope of this article; however, a basic approach is described.

Motor NCS of the MPN recorded at the AH with stimulation at the ankle and popliteal fossa are recommended. In addition, motor NCS of the LPN recorded at the FDMB can be performed. In patients with a significant degree of heel discomfort, this author often performs motor NCS of the ICN recorded at the ADQP.

The author also typically performs mixed NCS of the MPN and LPN by stimulating the sole of the foot and recording posterior to the medial malleolus. These mixed NCS have been shown to be more sensitive than the corresponding motor studies in patients with MPN or LPN neuropathies.[23] It should be noted, however, that mixed NCS may be challenging to obtain in the elderly or those with structural foot abnormalities. In patients with unilateral complaints, absence of the bilateral mixed NCS should be interpreted with caution. Bilateral alterations in these mixed NCS may represent an underlying peripheral polyneuropathy.[23,24] Again, these NCS findings should be combined with the other EDx results and the history and physical examination to provide meaningful interpretation.

MCN sensory NCS may be attempted in patients with altered heel sensation. However, the responses are small and can be technically challenging to perform. Again, absence of this response should be interpreted with caution.

The EDx data obtained from the tibial nerve branches can be compared against known normal values and often necessitate contralateral comparison. Comparison ipsilateral SPN and sural sensory and CPN motor studies are also warranted to exclude more diffuse involvement (**Fig. 2**, **Table 2**).

When attempting to differentiate which tibial nerve branches may be involved, EMG of the foot muscles is critical. At the minimum, EMG should include one muscle supplied by each of the tibial nerve motor branches. This author frequently performs EMG of the AH (supplied by MPN), the fourth DIP (supplied by the LPN), and the ADQP (supplied by the ICN). Also, comparison EMG evaluation of the ipsilateral EDB and more proximal tibial, peroneal, and sciatic supplied nerves is important to exclude more proximal disorders. EMG comparison of the contralateral tibial-supplied foot muscles may be performed to strengthen the electrodiagnostic evidence supporting a focal process.

### Sciatic Nerve

Much of the sciatic nerve anatomy and related NCS have been discussed in the peroneal and tibial nerve sections. Classically sciatic neuropathies present with sensory and motor disturbances in both the tibial and peroneal supplied territories. However, the peroneal fibers may be preferentially affected, leading to a clinical syndrome that appears to reflect a more purely peroneal pattern. Careful history and physical examination may help prove there are extraperoneal findings including foot inversion or knee flexion weakness and sural or plantar nerve sensory changes. Routine motor NCS of the tibial and peroneal nerves are warranted. Again, the peroneal motor NCS abnormalities may be more prominent than the tibial motor NCS findings. The ipsilateral sural and superficial peroneal sensory NCS should also be performed. Proof of more subtle sciatic nerve lesions and elimination of a more diffuse peripheral polyneuropathy may be assisted by comparison of these sensory NCS contralaterally. The saphenous nerve should be spared in sciatic neuropathies. Therefore, a normal saphenous sensory NCS would also help support evidence of a sciatic neuropathy.

EMG abnormalities in the peroneal and tibial supplied muscles should be expected in a sciatic neuropathy. More precise localization of the sciatic nerve lesion is assisted by EMG testing of the various sciatic-supplied hamstring muscles. If EMG abnormalities are found in the gluteal muscles, lumbosacral paraspinals, or other nonsciatic-supplied muscles, a plexopathy or radiculopathy etiology should be considered.

## LUMBOSACRAL RADICULOPATHY AND PLEXOPATHY

Lumbosacral radiculopathy and less commonly plexopathy may present as distal lower extremity symptoms. It is important to consider degenerative disc or joint

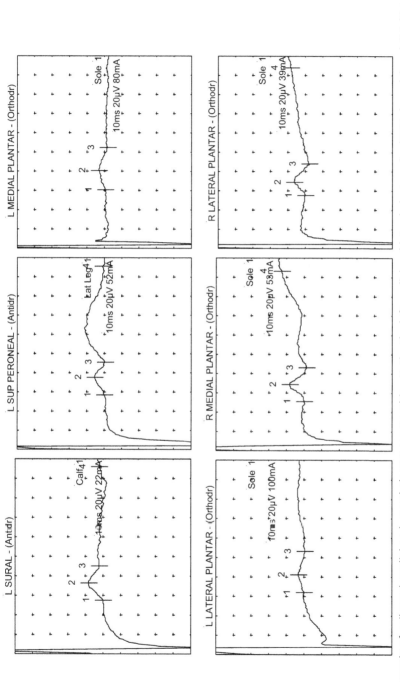

**Fig. 2.** Example of unilateral medial and ateral plantar neuropathies. Notice the left medial and lateral plantar mixed NCS show delayed distal latencies with decreased amplitudes, especial γ on contralateral comparison. The ipsilateral sural and superficial peroneal sensory NCS are normal.

**Table 2**
**Mixed and sensory nerve conduction study findings**

| Nerve/Sites | Rec. Site | Onset Lat ms | Peak Lat ms | NP Amp μV | PP Amp μV | Segments | Distance cm | Velocity m/s | Area μVms |
|---|---|---|---|---|---|---|---|---|---|
| L Sural-(Antidr) | | | | | | | | | |
| Calf | Lat Mall | 2.75 | 3.65 | 17.9 | 13.5 | Calf-Lat Mall | 14 | 50.9 | 14.5 |
| L Sup Peroneal-(Antidr) | | | | | | | | | |
| Lat Leg | Ankle | 2.85 | 3.75 | 12.3 | 12.6 | Lat Leg–Ankle | 14 | 49.1 | 10.8 |
| L Medial Plantar-(Orthodr) | | | | | | | | | |
| Sole | Med Mall | 3.05 | **4.05** | **7.4** | 9.7 | Sole-Med Mall | 14 | 45.9 | 10.1 |
| R Medial Plantar-(Orthodr) | | | | | | | | | |
| Sole | Med Mall | 2.55 | 3.45 | 16.5 | 19.1 | Sole-Med Mall | 14 | 54.9 | 13.6 |
| L Lateral Plantar-(Orthodr) | | | | | | | | | |
| Sole | Med Mall | 3.20 | **4.10** | **6.5** | 7.5 | Sole-Med Mall | 14 | 43.8 | 7.6 |
| R Lateral Plantar-(Orthodr) | | | | | | | | | |
| Sole | Med Mall | 2.75 | 3.45 | 12.3 | 17.0 | Sole-Med Mall | 14 | 50.9 | 12.6 |

*Abbreviations:* Amp, amplitude; Antidr, antidromic; cm, centimeter; L, left; Lat, lateral; Mall, malleolus; Med, medial; ms, milliseconds; m/s, meters/second; Orthodr, orthodromic; NP, negative to peak; Onset Lat, onset latency; Peak Lat, peak latency; PP, peak to peak; R, right; Rec, recording; μV, microvolt.

disease as a potential source of foot complaints given the relative frequency of these disorders. Although many patients have a history of low back pain, they may be dismissive of their back pain given its chronic nature, or they may not relate it to their foot symptoms. In addition, some patients with interspinal pathology do not have significant back pain.

Routine motor and sensory NCS as described in the sciatic section of this article may be performed when evaluating for more proximal lesions. In mild cases of lumbosacral radiculopathy, all NCS are frequently normal. The sensory NCS should be normal, since radiculopathic processes typically occur proximal to the DRG as previously described. If present, sensory NCS abnormalities would point toward a primary process distal to the DRG such as a plexopathy or other peripheral nerve lesion.[1] SNAP changes could also be present in patients with radiculopathy with an overlapping peripheral nerve process. Careful consideration must be given to all of these clinical possibilities.

Routine motor NCS of the lower extremities are recorded over the foot muscles supplied by the lower lumbosacral nerve roots. Additionally, a significant degree of axon loss must occur before CMAP amplitudes fall outside of the normal range. Therefore, only more advanced cases of L5, S1, or S2 radiculopathy will show CMAP changes on routine motor NCS.

The EMG examination, however, is more sensitive for axonal loss changes than the CMAP amplitude. EMG is particularly important in EDx evaluation of radiculopathies and plexopathies. EMG can demonstrate abnormalities in muscles not easily accessible by NCS. This is especially significant given the importance of examining the proximal leg musculature in suspected lumbosacral radiculopathy or plexopathy. A radiculopathy is suggested by EMG abnormalities present in at least 2 muscles with different peripheral nerve supply, but the same spinal root innervation, including the corresponding paraspinal muscles. Furthermore, EMG is expected to be normal in muscles supplied by the adjacent unaffected myotomes.[1] For example, increased IA, PSW, and polyphasic MUAP in the peroneus longus, medial gastrocnemius, gluteus maximus, and lower lumbosacral paraspinals muscles, with normal tibialis anterior and vastus medialis muscles, is most consistent with a L5-S1 radiculopathy. Alternatively, if the lumbosacral paraspinals were normal and the corresponding SNAPs were abnormal, this would suggest the presence of a lumbosacral plexopathy. A similar example of a unilateral L5 radiculopathy is shown in **Table 3**.

## PERIPHERAL POLYNEUROPATHY

While there are many types of polyneuropathies, the most common pattern for a peripheral polyneuropathy (PPN) involves a distal symmetric length-dependent process. This results in initial symptoms in the distal feet that may eventually progress to the classic stocking and glove pattern. The sensory and motor nerves in the feet will be most likely to reflect abnormalities on physical and EDx examination.[25] The EDx examination for a suspected PPN should at the minimum include sural sensory and peroneal motor NCS.[7] However, recent studies have shown that abnormalities in the mixed plantar NCS may be the most sensitive indicators of distal PPN.[23,24] However, these mixed plantar NCS studies may have technical limitations as previously described. If a PPN involving large nerve fibers is present, sensory or motor NCS may show evidence of decreased conduction velocity, delayed distal latency, or decreased amplitude in multiple peripheral nerves. Of note, small fiber nerves are not evaluated by routine NCS/EMG testing; therefore purely small fiber PPN cannot be excluded with the EDx studies as described.

**Table 3**
**Example electromyography findings of a right L5 radiculopathy**

EMG Summary Table

| | Spontaneous | | | | | | MUAP | | | Recruitment | |
|---|---|---|---|---|---|---|---|---|---|---|---|
| | IA | PSW | Fibs | SSFD Size | Fasic | Other | Amplitude | Duration | Complexity | Pattern | Frequency |
| R. TIB Anterior | Increased | 2+ | None | 200–400 µV | None | None | Normal | Increased | Mild polyphasia | Normal | Normal |
| R. Gastrocn (Med) | Normal | None | None | N/A | None | None | Normal | Normal | Normal | Normal | Normal |
| R. Tibialis Posterior | Increased | 2+ | None | 200–400 µV | None | None | Normal | Increased | Mild polyphasia | Normal | Normal |
| R. Vast Medialis | Normal | None | None | N/A | None | None | Normal | Normal | Normal | Normal | Normal |
| R. Peron Longus | Increased | 2+ | None | 200–400 µV | None | None | Normal | Increased | Mild polyphasia | Normal | Normal |
| R. Add Longus | Normal | None | None | N/A | None | None | Normal | Normal | Normal | Normal | Normal |
| R. Gluteus Med | Increased | 2+ | 1+ | 200–400 µV | None | None | Normal | Increased | Mild polyphasia | Normal | Normal |
| R. Lumb PSP (M/L) | Increased | 2+ | 1+ | 200–400 µV | None | None | — | — | — | — | — |

Tabular data for the needle EMG data are shown. Note the findings of increased insertional activity (IA), abnormal spontaneous activity (Fibs and PSW), and motor unit morphology changes in the limb and paraspinal muscles that receive supply from the L5 myotome. Also note that these same limb muscles have different peripheral nerve supply (peroneal, tibial, and superior gluteal). The muscles that do not have a dominant supply from the L5 myotome are normal.

*Abbreviations*: Add, Adductor; Fibs, fibrillation potentials; Gastrocn (Med), gastrocnemius (Medial); Lumb PSP (M/L), lumbar paraspinals (middle/lower); Med, Medius; MUAP, motor unit action potentials; Peron, peroneus; PSW, positive sharp waves; R, right; SSFD, spontaneous single fiber discharges; Tib, Tibialis; Vast, vastus; µV, microvolts.

The combination of NCS findings seen can help distinguish whether the PPN is primarily demyelinative or axonal in nature. This distinction may help narrow the differential diagnosis when seeking the PPN's etiology. A PPN with axonal features may show EMG evidence of Fibs or PSW in the distal foot and leg muscles but not in more proximal muscles supplied by the same peripheral nerves. Given the distal distribution of the most common type of PPN, care should be taken to rule out a PPN when the EDx evidence is suggestive of bilateral distal tibial neuropathies. In addition to the previously mentioned NCS testing, EMG of the EDB or extensor hallicus longus may be helpful in these cases.[14]

## SUMMARY

There are many peripheral nerve abnormalities that can result in common foot and ankle complaints. The electrodiagnostic medicine consultation can be extremely helpful in differentiating the etiology of a patient's symptoms and thus directing further clinical care. The electrodiagnostic study is a supplement to the history and physical examination, and all elements should be thoughtfully incorporated to provide a clinically meaningful interpretation of the electrical data. Detailed knowledge and careful consideration of the anatomy and technical aspects of electrodiagnosis are critical in evaluation of lower extremity neurogenic problems.

## REFERENCES

1. Dumitru D, Zwarts MJ. Radiculopathies and focal peripheral neuropathies. In: Dumitru D, Amato A, Zwarts MJ, editors. Electrodiagnostic medicine. Philadelphia: Hanley and Belfus; 2002. p. 713–75, 1043–106.
2. Asp JP, Rand JA. Peroneal nerve palsy after total knee arthroplasty. Clin Orthop Relat Res 1990;261:233–7.
3. Noble J, Munro CA, Prasad VS, et al. Analysis of upper and lower extremity peripheral nerve injuries in a population of patients with multiple trauma. J Trauma 1998;45:116–22.
4. Pickett JB. Localizing peroneal nerve lesions to the knee by motor conduction studies. Arch Neurol 1984;41:192–5.
5. Gesini L, Jandolo B, Pietrangeli A. The anterior tarsal tunnel syndrome. J Bone Joint Surg Am 1984;66:786–7.
6. Borges L, Haller M, Selkoe D, et al. The anterior tarsal syndrome: report of two cases. J Neurosurg 1981;54:89–92.
7. England JD, Gronseth GS, Franklin G, et al. Distal symmetrical polyneuropathy; definition for clinical research. Muscle Nerve 2005;31:113–23.
8. Spillane K, Nagendran K, Kunzru KM. Anomalous communication in the anterior tarsal tunnel syndrome. Muscle Nerve 1997;20:395–6.
9. Bergman RA, Thompson SA, Afifi AK. Catalog of human variation. Baltimore (MD): Urban & Schwarzenberg; 1984.
10. Andresen BL, Wertsch JJ, Stewart WA. Anterior tarsal tunnel syndrome. Arch Phys Med Rehabil 1992;73:1112–6.
11. Park TA, Del Toro DR. Electrodiagnostic evaluation of the foot. Phys Med Rehabil Clin N Am 1998;9:881–2.
12. Akita K, Sakamoto H, Sato T. Lateromedial and dorsoplantar borders among supplying areas of nerves innervating the intrinsic muscles of the foot. Anat Rec 1999;255(4):465–70.
13. Gatens PF, Saeed MA. Electromyographic findings in the intrinsic muscles of normal feet. Arch Phys Med Rehabil 1982;63:317–8.

14. Spindler HA, Reischer MA, Felsenthal G. Electrodiagnostic assessment in suspected tarsal tunnel syndrome. Phys Med Rehabil Clin N Am 1994;5:595–612.
15. Adkinson DP, Bosse MJ, Gaccione DR, et al. Anatomical variations in the course of the superficial peroneal nerve. J Bone Joint Surg Am 1991;73:112.
16. Styf J. Entrapment of the superficial peroneal nerve. Diagnosis and results of decompression. J Bone Joint Surg Br 1989;71:131–5.
17. Sridhara CR, Izzo KL. Terminal sensory branches of the superficial peroneal nerve: an entrapment syndrome. Arch Phys Med Rehabil 1985;66:789–91.
18. Gutmann L. Atypical deep peroneal neuropathy in the presence of accessory deep peroneal nerve. J Neurol Neurosurg Psychiatry 1970;33:453–6.
19. Blackshear BM, Lutz GE, Obrien SJ. Sural nerve entrapment after injury to the gastrocnemius: a case report. Arch Phys Med Rehabil 1999;80:604–5.
20. Ferkel RD, Heath DD, Guhl JF. Neurological complication of ankle arthroscopy. Arthroscopy 1996;12(2):200–8.
21. Dellon AL, Mackinnon SE. Tibial nerve branching in the tarsal tunnel. Arch Neurol 1984;41:645–6.
22. Havel PE, Ebraheim NA, Clark SE, et al. Tibial branching in the tarsal tunnel. Foot Ankle 1988;9:117–9.
23. Galardi G, Amadio S, Maderna L, et al. Electrophysiologic studies in tarsal tunnel syndrome: diagnostic reliability of motor distal latency, mixed nerve and sensory nerve conduction studies. Am J Phys Med Rehabil 1994;73:193–8.
24. Uluc K, Isak B, Borucu D, et al. Medial plantar and dorsal sural nerve conduction studies increased the sensitivity in the detection of neuropathy in diabetic patients. Clin Neurophysiol 2008;119:880–5.
25. Singleton JR. Evaluation and treatment of painful peripheral polyneuropathy. Semin Neurol 2005;25:185–95.

# Nerve Problems in the Lower Extremity

Wilson Z. Ray, MD[a], Susan E. Mackinnon, MD[b],*

**KEYWORDS**

- Lower extremity peripheral nerve injuries • Management
- Repair strategies • Autografts

The surgical treatment of peripheral nerve injuries has made significant advances since the turn of the century.[1] Improved microsurgical techniques, the widespread use of the operating microscope, and a greater understanding of peripheral nerve biology have dramatically improved functional outcomes. In addition, the recent use of nerve transfers along with advances in the understanding of the pathophysiology of nerve injury and regeneration has further provided the field with a period of rapid evolution.

Restoration of function following peripheral nerve injuries is directed toward rapid and complete reinnervation of distal motor endplates and sensory receptors while minimizing donor site morbidity. The degree of functional recovery following a nerve injury is dependent on several factors: time from injury, patient age, mechanism of injury, the proximity of the lesion to distal targets, and other associated soft tissue or vascular injuries.[2–4] Prompt repair of motor nerve injuries leads to improved outcomes by minimizing the time to motor endplate reinnervation.[5,6] Anecdotal experience suggests younger patients tend to exhibit a more robust regenerative capacity, with superior nerve regeneration following repair. The mechanism of injury is an important determinant of the longitudinal extent of the damage. It is known that proximal lesions require nerve regeneration to occur over longer distances, increasing the time to target end-organ reinnervation. Lastly, significant soft tissue or vascular injuries can result in scarring and distortion of the anatomy, which can complicate any plans for future repair.

## NERVE GAPS

When tension-free primary repair is not possible, a suitable alternative must be pursued. Nerve regeneration occurs in a very regulated and predictable fashion;

[a] Department of Neurological Surgery, Washington University School of Medicine, 660 South Euclid Avenue, St Louis, MO 63110, USA
[b] Division of Plastic and Reconstructive Surgery, Washington University School of Medicine, 660 South Euclid Avenue, St Louis, MO 63110, USA
* Corresponding author.
*E-mail address:* mackinnons@wustl.edu

Foot Ankle Clin N Am 16 (2011) 243–254
doi:10.1016/j.fcl.2011.01.009
1083-7515/11/$ – see front matter © 2011 Elsevier Inc. All rights reserved.

foot.theclinics.com

thus regardless of the repair strategy that is employed, the surgical technique is similar. The proximal and distal nerve stumps are cut back until normal fascicular structure is encountered (**Fig. 1**). This attention to the longitudinal extent of injury is critical to achieve a good functional outcome. If a repair is performed within the zone of injury (see **Fig. 1**A), regenerating axons be impeded by neuroma and scar tissue. Typically bread-loafing proximally and distally reveals about one centimeter of scar tissue before a normal fascicular pattern is noted. In the case of a failed primary repair, care must be taken to ensure that any graft is placed completely outside of the zone of injury while placing minimal tension on the repair site through the entire range of motion at the joint. In general, the authors have found that in the care of a pervious failed primary repair, a 4 cm nerve graft is usually required to ensure a tension-free repair outside of the zone of injury. In smaller diameter failed nerve repairs a shorter graft length is the norm.

A primary tenet of all repairs requires that all nerve repairs and reconstructions be performed in a tension-free manner. This allows for early postoperative movement and nerve gliding, thus minimizing scar adherence. In addition, a thorough understanding of nerve topography is also critical for any successful nerve repair. A misaligned repair could result in excellent regeneration but poor functional recovery if motor and sensory fascicles are not properly oriented. Lastly, is important to decompress or transpose nerves at known areas of adjacent or distal entrapment. As a nerve regenerates, it will often hold or stall in an area of known nerve compression (eg, peroneal nerve at the fibular head, the tibial nerve at the soleus arch, and the tarsal tunnel with proximal sciatic injury), reducing potential functional recovery.

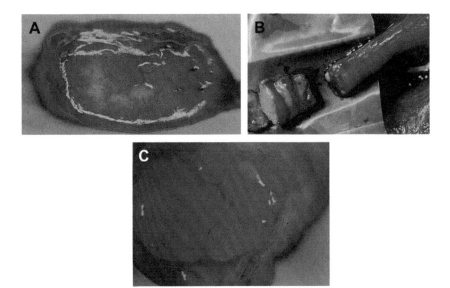

**Fig. 1.** (*A*) Photograph of resected neuroma with disruption of architecture. Sutures are evident from a previous repair. (*B*) Step-wise removal of scar tissue until healthy nerve fascicles are encountered. (*C*) Healthy nerve outside the zone of injury, depicting organized architecture with healthy fascicles before nerve grafting. (*Adapted from* Ray WZ, Mackinnon SE. Management of nerve gaps: autografts, allografts, nerve transfers, and end-to-side neurorrhaphy. Exp Neurol 2010;223(1):78; with permission from Elsevier.)

## Autogenous Nerve Grafts

The traditional gold standard for repair of segmental peripheral nerve injuries has relied upon autologous nerve grafts. Autogenous grafts act as a structurally inert scaffold for axonal regeneration, providing the necessary matrix, neurotrophic growth factors and viable Schwann cells (SCs). In all nerve repairs, the distal stump releases neurotrophic growth factors that guide the regenerating axons.[7–9] As opposed to acellular grafts, resident SCs in autografts provide support for subsequent remyelination, making proximal and distal SC migration unnecessary.[10]

Appropriate autogenous graft selection is dependent on few factors: the size of the nerve gap, caliber of graft required, location of proposed nerve repair, and associated donor-site morbidity. The sural nerve is the most commonly used autograft,[11] yet there are many other suitable alternatives, including:

The medial and lateral cutaneous nerves of the forearm
Dorsal cutaneous branch of the ulnar nerve
The greater auricular nerve
Superficial and deep peroneal nerves
Intercostal nerves
The posterior and lateral cutaneous nerves of the thigh.[12,13]

As previously discussed with nerve gaps and, when an interposition graft is used, it is critical to avoid any tension at the repair site.

There are several pros and cons for using nerve autografts. As mentioned, autografts provide a nonimmunogenic graft, with intact endoneurial tubes and viable resident SCs. In addition, they serve as a bridge to overcome irreducible nerve gaps. The drawbacks of autografts are: scarring, sensory/motor loss, neuroma formation, additional incision, and the inherent limited supply. A favorite nerve graft is the medial antebrachial cutaneous nerve (MABC). It can be harvested from the elbow to the axilla and has two potential branches. The distal end of the donor MABC nerve can be sewn end to side with or without an acellular graft to the adjacent MABC nerve if just one is needed or to the sensory side (lateral side) of the median nerve if the entire MABC is required.

## Nerve Allografts

In rare cases of severe global plexus or segmental nerve injuries, the use of donor-related or cadaveric nerve allografts can be considered. Like solid organs, nerve allografts require global immunosuppression and the associated morbidity of systemic immunosuppression. Unlike other tissue allotransplantation, immunosuppression is only required until donor SCs can be replaced by migrating host SCs (approximately 18–24 months). There are several techniques that have been used to reduce allograft antigenicity (eg, cold preservation, irradiation, or lyophilization).[14–23] The authors' clinical protocol is ABO matched donors, small-diameter donor nerves, cold preservation (4°–5°C for 7 days), 3 days of pretreatment with FK506, and continued immunosuppression until the Tinel sign has crossed the distal graft site.[24]

While SCs represent a critical component for nerve regeneration over long gaps, donor SCs serve a dual role following nerve allotransplantation. Donor SCs support remyelination until host SCs have migrated into the allograft. Donor SCs also represent the main antigenic target for host rejection, taking on the role of facultative antigen presenting cells. This dual role prevents complete removal of the donor SCs and simultaneously maintains the requirement for systemic immunosuppression.[25–31] Over time, host SCs will eventually replace donor SCs completely.

As the understanding and experience with nerve transfers has evolved, dependence on nerve allotransplantation has diminished. Despite the decreased use of nerve allografts clinically, nerve allografting and its role in composite tissue transplantation remain an area of keen interest. Unlike composite tissue transplantation, nerve allotransplantation requires only temporary immunosuppression. Once adequate host SC migration has occurred, systemic immunosuppression can be withdrawn. In addition, the currently used immunosuppressive agent (FK-506) has been shown to enhance neuroregeneration[32–34] and is being studied as a potential therapeutic agent for a more widespread application in all significant nerve injury patients.

Nerve allografts have several distinct advantages, including: potentially unlimited supply, being readily available, and avoiding donor site morbidity. The prohibitive drawback to nerve allotransplantation remains the morbidity associated with systemic immunosuppression.

### End-to-Side Coaptation

The concept of end-to-side coaptation is not a new one.[35,36] End-to-side coaptation represents an alternative in cases where there is no proximal nerve stump and the injured distal stump is coapted to the side of a donor nerve. End-to-side repair is dependent upon axonal sprouting from the intact donor nerve. Although the topic is still somewhat controversial, it has been demonstrated and is now fairly well accepted that sensory sprouting only requires an epineural window, yet motor regeneration requires some degree of axotomy. In 1999, Matsumoto and colleagues[37] demonstrated that although collateral sprouting occurs in the absence of donor nerve axotomy, only sensory reinnervation occurs. Hayashi and colleagues,[38] who designed an end-to-side coaptation rat model that preserved the donor nerve initially reported that even in the absence of donor nerve injury collateral sprouting occurs. However, when the experiment was repeated in a more sophisticated animal model, it was demonstrated that only sensory axons sprouted de novo without injury, while motor axons did not.[39] The authors' current clinical practice has yielded excellent results with low morbidity using well-planned nerve transfers, and the authors generally limit the use of end-to-side repairs to reconstruction of noncritical sensory deficits[24] or to restore some sensation back into a donor nerve territory as described previously.

End-to-side repair is a useful strategy when only sensory recovery is required, but it can be applied to motor regeneration when an axotomy is performed.[40] The biggest obstacle for widespread use for motor regeneration is the requirement for motor axotomy.

### Nerve Conduits

While significant clinical and laboratory efforts have been invested into the development of a viable nerve conduit, the current clinical applications remain fairly limited. The authors limit their use of nerve conduits to the repair of noncritical small diameter sensory nerves, gaps less than 3 cm, and as a nerve repair wrap.[24] In general in the authors' practice, acellularized allografts have largely been replaced by nerve conduits. The authors believe the combination of intact endoneurial tubes, combined with sufficient levels of neurotrophic factors, is critical for meaningful nerve regeneration. It is important to understand that if the volume of a conduit increases beyond a critical diameter (**Fig. 2**), regeneration will not occur unless the length of the conduit is appropriately shortened.

The pros of nerve conduits are: avoiding donor site morbidity, unlimited supply, and ready availability. Conduits have several important limitations: lack of endoneurial tubes and SCs, limited to short nerve gaps (<3 cm), and variable outcomes.

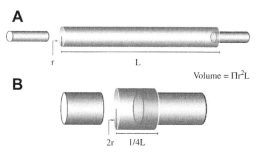

**Fig. 2.** Illustrates the importance of diameter in the volume of a nerve gap. The formula for volume is $V = \Pi r^2 L$, thus doubling the radius (conduit *B*) requires a length ¼ of conduit *A* to maintain an equal volume. *Abbreviations:* L, length; $\Pi$ = pi (~3.14); r, radius; V, volume. (*From* Moore AM, Kasukurthi R, Magill CK, et al. Limitations of conduits in peripheral nerve repairs. Hand (NY) 2009;4(2):180–6; with permission.)

## Nerve Transfers

While the use of nerve transfers for brachial plexus injuries and upper extremity nerve reconstructions is now well established, the widespread use of nerve transfers for lower extremity repairs is far more limited.[41–45] Although there are no definitive guidelines for the use of nerve transfers in general, the authors use the following set of indications: brachial plexus injuries or other proximal injuries, long distance from target motor end plates, delayed presentation, significant limb trauma resulting in segmental loss of nerve function, and previous injury with significant scarring around vital bony or vascular structures.

With all transfers, when selecting the appropriate donor nerves several criteria must be considered: proximity of donor nerve to the recipient nerve motor end plates, availability of redundant or expendable donor nerve, synergism of donor muscles to target muscles, similarity in number of motor or sensory axons between donor and recipient nerves, and size matching. The authors in the past performed 6 tibial-to-peroneal motor nerve transfers and were not impressed that patients could voluntarily dorsiflex the ankle. Currently the authors believe that a tibial tendon transfer is superior to a nerve transfer for peroneal nerve palsy with long peroneal nerve injuries or prolonged denervation times.

The benefits of nerve transfers include: avoiding donor autograft harvest and the associated morbidity and providing earlier reinnervation to target motor endplates.

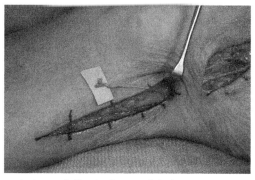

**Fig. 3.** Intraoperative photograph illustrating medial plantar nerve neurolysis and proximal transfer.

**A**                                          Pain Questionnaire

Name: _____          Date: _____

Age: _____ Sex: Male___ Female___ Dominant Hand: Right___ Left ___ Diagnosis: _____

1.  Pain is difficult to describe. Circle the words that best describe your symptoms:

| Burning | Throbbing | Aching | Stabbing | Tingling | Twisting | Squeezing |
|---------|-----------|--------|----------|----------|----------|-----------|
| Cramping | Cutting | Shooting | Numbing | Vague | Stinging | Indescribable |
| Pulling | Smarting | Pressure | Coldness | Dull | Other: _____ | |

Level of symptoms: place a mark through the line to indicate the level of your pain, if zero is no pain and the end of the line is the most severe pain you can imagine having.

2.  Mark your average level of pain in the last month

    No Pain                                          Most Severe Pain

3.  Mark your worst level of pain in the last week

Right    No Pain                                          Most Severe Pain

Left     No Pain                                          Most Severe Pain

4.  Where is your pain? (Draw on diagram)

R                        L  L                        R

Mark on this scale how your pain has affected your quality of life:

0%                                          100%
Very little                              A large amount

**Fig. 4.** (A) Pain evaluation. This form is given to each patient on every visit, which is useful for both an objective measure of pain, localization of pain, and a record to refer to postoperatively. (B) Pain evaluation specifically for patients with lower extremity pain.

The drawbacks include the potential loss of function from donor nerves and the fact that the donor muscle is no longer a suitable donor for future muscle transfers.

### Nerves of the lower extremity
The authors believe that peroneal nerve compression is relatively unrecognized. The three entrapment points that they see are the common peroneal nerve at the fibular

**B**

Name:_____        Date:_____

RIGHT

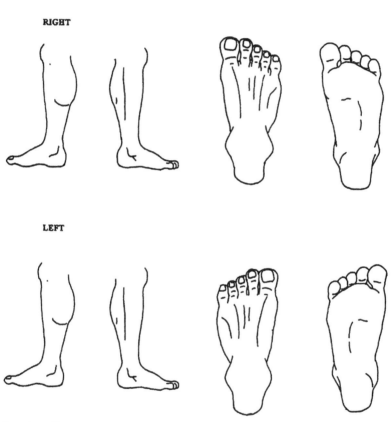

LEFT

**Fig. 4.** *(continued)*

head, the superficial peroneal nerve in the leg, and the deep peroneal on the dorsum of the foot. The authors use both a localizing Tinel signs and positive scratch collapse to determine which are most symptomatic. Scratch collapse is a useful objective test that does not rely on the patient's report of pain, but rather uses the brief loss of muscle tone if a patient does in fact have allodynia due to compression neuropathy.[46] In addition, the authors have seen situations where patients have compression at the fibular head and over time, the nerve regenerates and becomes entrapped more distally over the superficial peroneal or over the dorsum of the foot. Patients present with recurrent symptoms of pain and sensory disturbances, and a more distal release will improve these symptoms. When the authors perform decompressions for pain, they always advise the patients at discharge after common peroneal nerve release, if they have recurrent pain months or years later, then they should consider returning to see whether there is a distal entrapment that could be released in the superficial or deep peroneal entrapment points.

In regards to the tibial nerve compression at the tarsal tunnel, the authors recommend the use of two incisions, one over the tibial nerve and one more distally over the plantar tunnels. The authors take care to release the distal medial and lateral plantar tunnels, and frequently release a bit of plantar fascia distally. The cutaneous branch from the medial plantar nerve innervates the medial sole of the foot and can be injured with surgery or with plantar surgeries; if this is the case, the authors neurolyze it and transfer it proximally (**Fig. 3**). The authors also release more proximally, more now than they did in the past to make sure that the fascia in the distal leg is not compressing the nerve. Another point is that in patients after tarsal tunnel who still have symptoms in the plantar aspect of the foot, the authors look for a proximal entrapment point at the tendinous leading edge of the soleus muscle. They identify this by the lack of pain with deep palpation along the course of the tibial nerve in the normal calf as compared with pain exactly at the point where the tibial nerve goes underneath the soleus arch in the symptomatic leg. Notably, the scratch collapse test is not useful in determining nerve compression at the soleus arch, probably because the nerve is deep. By contrast, it is very useful for tarsal tunnel and is as useful for tarsal tunnel as a Tinel sign. The authors also pay close attention to patients who have significant pronation of their ankle, as a release will take pressure off the nerve, but if the pronation is not corrected, then the patients are still putting stretch on the tibial nerve that a tarsal tunnel release will not address.

In regards to neuromas in the foot and ankle, the pain drawing (**Fig. 4**) and the patient's description of the distribution of his or her pain are helpful in determining what nerves are involved. The authors will specifically look for Tinel signs proximal to the area of a potential painful scar and neuroma, as a proximal positive Tinel can help to identify what nerve is involved. The proximal Tinel sign represents the misdirected axons from the neuroma that have regenerated proximally. Sometimes tapping over the area where the patient has maximum pain is not helpful, because it is just too painful for the patient. Therefore a proximal Tinel sign can often be useful, because it is less painful. With the saphenous nerve, the authors will frequently block the potentially involved nerve to see if that helps relieve pain. When possible, the authors try to reconstruct the small cutaneous nerves such as superficial peroneal with an acellularized allograft. If this is unsuccessful, the authors will proximally transfer the nerve and use a cautery and crush paradigm (**Fig. 5**) and transfer the nerve proximally. For the superficial peroneal, the authors make sure they also do a fasciotomy to fully release

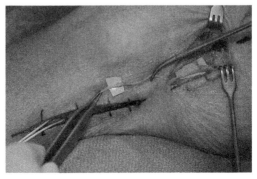

**Fig. 5.** Intraoperative photograph depicts the creation an axonotmetic injury.

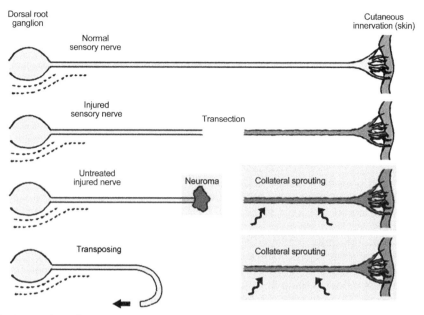

**Fig. 6.** Creation of an axonotometic injury prevents the brain from perceiving a neurotmetic injury and avoids leaving denervated territories unsatisfied.

the nerve from its entrapment fascia, so that there is no increased pressure on the distal end of the nerve within a tight myofascial compartment. In a situation with, for example, a sural neuroma, the authors would treat it in the same way, moving the nerve proximally; however, if there is irritation on the superficial peroneal nerve, then they would recommend decompression of that nerve at its entrapment site. With the sural nerve, the authors will frequently see development of peroneal nerve irritation after treating the sural nerve. In these cases, a release of the superficial peroneal nerve through its entrapment point frequently will relieve that pain. Finally, dorsal column stimulators can be very useful with foot and ankle pain resistant to surgical intervention.

With Morton's neuroma, the author's general philosophy will be to decompress the plantar digital nerve through a dorsal approach, telling the patient that if that is not successful, then they would use a dorsal approach to remove the neuroma and with microbipolar cautery, cauterize the distal portion of the plantar digital nerve. If that does not work or when there is recurrent/persistent pain, the authors will use a plantar approach. They cap the distal end with microbipolar cautery, clamp it proximally to crush it so as to make an axonotmetic injury (see **Fig. 5**) so that the brain is perceiving first an axonotmetic injury, not the neurotmetic injury, and then transfer this very far distally to avoid leaving denervated territories unsatisfied (**Fig. 6**).

## SUMMARY

The use of different repair strategies is largely patient driven; careful attention to individual patient factors and realistic outcome goals facilitate a directed surgical approach. While each repair strategy offers its own set of pros and cons, the best course of action is determined by injury type, patient characteristics, and surgeon preferences.

## REFERENCES

1. Naff NJ, Ecklund JM. History of peripheral nerve surgery techniques. Neurosurg Clin N Am 2001;12(1):197–209.
2. Slutsky DA. Vincent peripheral nerve surgery. Philadelphia: Churchill Livingstone, Elsevier; 2006.
3. Gilbert A, Pivato G, Kheiralla T. Long-term results of primary repair of brachial plexus lesions in children. Microsurgery 2006;26(4):334–42.
4. Hentz VR, Narakas A. The results of microneurosurgical reconstruction in complete brachial plexus palsy. Assessing outcome and predicting results. Orthop Clin North Am 1988;19(1):107–14.
5. Tung TH, Mackinnon SE. Nerve transfers: indications, techniques, and outcomes. J Hand Surg Am 2010;35(2):332–41.
6. Kobayashi J, Mackinnon SE, Watanabe O, et al. The effect of duration of muscle denervation on functional recovery in the rat model. Muscle Nerve 1997;20(7): 858–66.
7. Brushart TM, Seiler 4th WA. Selective reinnervation of distal motor stumps by peripheral motor axons. Exp Neurol 1987;97(2):289–300.
8. Mackinnon SE, Dellon AL, Lundborg G, et al. A study of neurotrophism in a primate model. J Hand Surg Am 1986;11(6):888–94.
9. Lundborg G, Dahlin LB, Danielsen N, et al. Tissue specificity in nerve regeneration. Scand J Plast Reconstr Surg 1986;20(3):279–83.
10. Fukaya K, Hasegawa M, Mashitani T, et al. Oxidized galectin-1 stimulates the migration of Schwann cells from both proximal and distal stumps of transected nerves and promotes axonal regeneration after peripheral nerve injury. J Neuropathol Exp Neurol 2003;62(2):162–72.
11. Schlosshauer B, Dreesmann L, Schaller HE, et al. Synthetic nerve guide implants in humans: a comprehensive survey. Neurosurgery 2006;59(4):740–7 [discussion: 747–48].
12. Norkus T, Norkus M, Ramanauskas T. Donor, recipient, and nerve grafts in brachial plexus reconstruction: anatomical and technical features for facilitating the exposure. Surg Radiol Anat 2005;27(6):524–30.
13. Mackinnon SE, Dellon LE. Surgery of the peripheral nerve, vol. 1. 1st edition. New York Thieme; 1988.
14. Marmor L. The repair of peripheral nerves by irradiated homografts. Clin Orthop Relat Res 1964;34:161–9.
15. Campbell JB, Bassett AL, Boehler J. Frozen-irradiated homografts shielded with microfilter sheaths in peripheral nerve surgery. J Trauma 1963;3:303–11.
16. Hiles RW. Freeze-dried irradiated nerve homograft: a preliminary report. Hand 1972;4(1):79–84.
17. Anderson PN, Turmaine M. Peripheral nerve regeneration through grafts of living and freeze-dried CNS tissue. Neuropathol Appl Neurobiol 1986;12(4):389–99.
18. Wilhelm K, Ross A. Homeoplastic nerve transplantation with lyophilized nerve. Arch Orthop Unfallchir 1972;72(2):156–67.
19. Wilhelm K. Briding of nerve defects using lyophilized homologous grafts. Handchirurgie 1972;4(1):25–30.
20. Singh R, Lange SA. Experience with homologous lyophilised nerve grafts in the treatment of peripheral nerve injuries. Acta Neurochir (Wien) 1975;32(1–2):125–30.
21. Martini AK. The lyophilized homologous nerve graft for the prevention of neuroma formation (animal experiment study). Handchir Mikrochir Plast Chir 1985;17(5): 266–9.

22. Evans PJ, Mackinnon SE, Best TJ, et al. Regeneration across preserved peripheral nerve grafts. Muscle Nerve 1995;18(10):1128–38.
23. Lawson GM, Glasby MA. A comparison of immediate and delayed nerve repair using autologous freeze-thawed muscle grafts in a large animal model. The simple injury. J Hand Surg Br 1995;20(5):663–700.
24. Ray WZ, Mackinnon SE. Management of nerve gaps: autografts, allografts, nerve transfers, and end-to-side neurorrhaphy. Exp Neurol 2010;223(1):77–85.
25. Gulati AK. Immune response and neurotrophic factor interactions in peripheral nerve transplants. Acta Haematol 1998;99(3):171–4.
26. Gulati AK, Cole GP. Nerve graft immunogenicity as a factor determining axonal regeneration in the rat. J Neurosurg 1990;72(1):114–22.
27. Pollard JD, Gye RS, McLeod JG. An assessment of immunosuppressive agents in experimental peripheral nerve transplantation. Surg Gynecol Obstet 1971; 132(5):839–45.
28. Trumble TE, Shon FG. The physiology of nerve transplantation. Hand Clin 2000; 16(1):105–22.
29. Lassner F, Schaller E, Steinhoff G, et al. Cellular mechanisms of rejection and regeneration in peripheral nerve allografts. Transplantation 1989;48(3):386–92.
30. Mackinnon S, Hudson A, Falk R, et al. Nerve allograft response: a quantitative immunological study. Neurosurgery 1982;10(1):61–9.
31. Yu LT, Rostami A, Silvers WK, et al. Expression of major histocompatibility complex antigens on inflammatory peripheral nerve lesions. J Neuroimmunol 1990;30:121–8.
32. Gold BG, Katoh K, Storm-Dickerson T. The immunosuppressant FK506 increases the rate of axonal regeneration in rat sciatic nerve. J Neurosci 1995;15(11): 7509–16.
33. Feng FY, Ogden MA, Myckatyn TM, et al. FK506 rescues peripheral nerve allografts in acute rejection. J Neurotrauma 2001;18(2):217–29.
34. Mackinnon SE, Doolabh VB, Novak CB, et al. Clinical outcome following nerve allograft transplantation. Plast Reconstr Surg 2001;107(6):1419–29.
35. Balance C, Balance HA, Stewart P. Remarks on the operative treatment of chronic facial palsy of the peripheral origin. Br J Med 1903;2:1009–13.
36. Harris WaL VW. On the importance of accurate muscular analysis in lesions of the brachial plexus and the treatment of Erb's palsy and infantile paralysis of the upper extremity by cross-union of the nerve roots. Br Med J 1903;2: 1035.
37. Matsumoto M, Hirata H, Nishiyama M, et al. Schwann cells can induce collateral sprouting from intact axons. experimental study of end-to-side neurorrhaphy using a Y-chamber model. J Reconstr Microsurg 1999;15(4):281–6.
38. Hayashi A, Yanai A, Komuro Y, et al. Collateral sprouting occurs following end-to-side neurorrhaphy. Plast Reconstr Surg 2004;114(1):129–37.
39. Hayashi A, Pannucci C, Moradzadeh A, et al. Axotomy or compression is required for axonal sprouting following end-to-side neurorrhaphy. Exp Neurol 2008;211(2):539–50.
40. Ray WZ, Kasukurthi R, Yee A, et al. Functional recovery following an end to side neurorrhaphy of the accessory nerve to the suprascapular nerve: case report. Hand (NY) 2009. [Epub ahead of print].
41. Campbell AA, Eckhauser FE, Belzberg A, et al. Obturator nerve transfer as an option for femoral nerve repair: case report. Neurosurgery 2010;66:375 [discussion: 375].

42. Flores LP. Proximal motor branches from the tibial nerve as direct donors to restore function of the deep fibular nerve for treatment of high sciatic nerve injuries: a cadaveric feasibility study. Neurosurgery 2009;65(Suppl 6):218–24 [discussion 224–15].

43. Oppenheim JS, Spitzer DE, Winfree CJ. Spinal cord bypass surgery using peripheral nerve transfers: review of translational studies and a case report on its use following complete spinal cord injury in a human. Experimental article. Neurosurg Focus 2009;26(2):E6.

44. Bodily KD, Spinner RJ, Bishop AT. Restoration of motor function of the deep fibular (peroneal) nerve by direct nerve transfer of branches from the tibial nerve: an anatomical study. Clin Anat 2004;17(3):201–5.

45. Koshima I, Nanba Y, Tsutsui T, et al. Deep peroneal nerve transfer for established plantar sensory loss. J Reconstr Microsurg 2003;19(7):451–4.

46. Cheng CJ, Mackinnon-Patterson B, Beck JL, et al. Scratch collapse test for evaluation of carpal and cubital tunnel syndrome. J Hand Surg Am 2008;33(9): 1518–24.

# Peripheral Nerve Entrapments of the Lower Leg, Ankle, and Foot

Ryan M. Flanigan, MD, Benedict F. DiGiovanni, MD*

**KEYWORDS**

- Nerve entrapment • Peripheral nerve • Foot pain
- Anterior tarsal tunnel

Peripheral nerve entrapments of the lower extremity are a relatively rare and heterogeneous group of nerve disorders encompassing a wide variety of etiologies as well as clinical presentations. Such conditions often present a diagnostic challenge because of the diversity of patient presentations. As such, it is widely believed that these conditions are both underdiagnosed and underreported in the literature. Treatment for peripheral nerve entrapment is highly dependent upon proper identification of the involved nerve and determination of the anatomic location of compression. Fortunately, improvements to electrodiagnostic and imaging modalities have helped ease the previous near-total reliance on patient history and physical examination in diagnosis of these conditions. This determination allows one to choose the optimal treatment strategy tailored to the patient's individual pathology. In this article, we examine peripheral nerve entrapments in the lower extremity involving the sural, saphenous and common, superficial, and deep peroneal nerves. This article reviews the anatomy of the lower extremity as it relates to the course and common areas of entrapment for these nerves, illustrates characteristics of common presentations of each disorder, and examines operative and nonoperative options for treatment based on the best available evidence. A precise understanding of the anatomic course and motor/sensory distribution of each nerve, as well as recognition of the common areas of compression will aid in the correct diagnosis and optimal treatment for these disorders.

The authors have nothing to disclose.
Department of Orthopaedics, University of Rochester Medical Center, 601 Elmwood Avenue, Box 665, Rochester, NY 14642, USA
* Corresponding author.
*E-mail address:* Benedict_DiGiovanni@urmc.rochester.edu

## OVERVIEW OF NERVE ENTRAPMENT

Nerve entrapment is broadly defined as the compression or entrapment of a nerve as it passes through or by another anatomic structure, most commonly a fibro-osseous tunnel or fascial opening. Entrapment can occur through any of a number of mechanisms, which can be broadly grouped into internal or external factors. In addition, there are many medical conditions, particularly those leading to whole-body fluid accumulation, increased extracellular matrix production, or chronic inflammatory conditions that can cause nerve compressions. Thus, some nerve entrapments are directly related to the underlying condition and subsequently resolve as the offending condition is addressed. Optimal treatment for these patients, in many cases, is medical rather than surgical.

Although the entirety of the nerve appears compressed to the eye, microscopically the nerve fibers are not universally affected by compression. Superficially located fibers (the large diameter, heavily myelinated fibers such as light touch and motor fibers) tend to exhibit increased amounts of compression, while the deeper fibers (less myelinated fibers such as pain fibers) typically are less affected. Studies have shown that the area of greatest mechanical deformation occurs both in the superficial area of the nerve, as well as in the zone between compressed and uncompressed segments.[1] External pressures of 20 to 30 mm Hg have been shown to impair venular flow in the epineurium and to slow axonal transport. Pressures of 30 mm Hg result in changes to the permeability of these intraneural blood vessels, resulting in further increases of intraneural interstitial fluid pressure.[2] Experimentally induced higher pressures (130 to 150 mm Hg) resulted in an acute block to conduction[3] and resulted in changes in the morphology of nerve fibers, causing both epineural and perineural thickening and rapid loss of nerve function.[4] This provides a basic science basis for the common clinical observation that less "significant" nerve compression lasting shorter durations of time will more often result in quick recovery of function after decompression. In contrast, more "significant" nerve compressions of longer durations are more likely to require longer periods to restoration of function, or incomplete restoration of function, after decompression. Furthermore, these physiologic changes, particularly to the blood supply to the nerve, occur rapidly. Within hours edema can be seen in histologic samples, and within days and continuing for weeks there is inflammation, fibrin deposition, and axonal degeneration.[5]

### Stages/Classification

Nerve compression often progresses through a series of stages, with characteristic symptomology related to both the duration and the degree of compression. Mild and brief compression, such as occurs when a limb "falls asleep," produces an interruption in axoplasmic flow. No major structural changes or damage occurs, and the nerve normalizes when pressure is relieved. In severe, acute compression there is often a sequential invagination of the myelin sheath seen on microscopy. As compression becomes chronic, segmental demyelination is seen, resulting in slowed conduction of action potentials and distal Wallerian degeneration of the nerve.

There are 3 described clinical stages in ongoing nerve compression in patients. Stage I is characterized by intermittent paresthesias and sensory deficits occurring primarily at night. Stage II occurs after continued progressive compression, which leads to more severe and consistent symptoms (such as paresthesias, numbness, impaired dexterity, and so forth) that fail to resolve during the day. Stage III is defined as altered nerve microcirculation and edema leading to pronounced morphologic changes including segmental demyelination. This results in more constant pain that does not disappear, even if pressure is resolved.[6] Generally, Stage I conditions can be treated nonoperatively with therapy, brace wear, pain/inflammation control, and so forth. Stages II and III will more often result in surgical intervention.

## Sural Nerve Entrapment

The sural nerve is the most extensively studied nerve in humans because of its status as a purely sensory nerve and resultant frequent use as a nerve graft.[7]

### Anatomy

The sural nerve is a sensory nerve providing sensation to the posterolateral aspect of the distal one-third of the leg and the lateral border of the foot. In approximately 80% of the population, it arises from the distal union of the medial sural cutaneous branch of the tibial nerve and the peroneal communicating branch of the common peroneal nerve. Notably, the peroneal communicating branch is absent in about 20% of patients and thus the nerve is essentially a branch of the medial sural cutaneous nerve.[8] The nerve begins distal to the popliteal fossa, traveling between the heads of the gastrocnemius and pierces the deep fascia in the middle third of the posterior surface of the leg. At this point, it typically is joined by the peroneal communicating branch. It then continues down the posterolateral side of the leg, traversing distally along the lateral border of the Achilles tendon. A branch may be directly adjacent to the lateral border of the tendo Achilles as well as the main nerve usually found midway between the lateral edge of the tendo Achilles and the posterior border of the lateral malleolus. At this level, branches emerge to form the lateral calcaneal branches, which provide sensation to the lateral aspect of the heel. It next passes plantar to the lateral malleolus and posterior to the peroneal tendons, then curving anteriorly, traveling on the lateral border of the foot where it becomes the lateral dorsal cutaneous nerve of the foot.[9] As this nerve courses distally it usually divides at the base of the fifth metatarsal to form dorsal and plantar branches. The dorsal branch gives rise to the dorsal digital nerve to the lateral side of the fifth toe, and often will either provide innervation or anastamose with other digital nerves supplying the medial border of the fifth toe and lateral border of the fourth toe. The plantar branch provides sensibility along the lateral border distally and may join the distal branches of the lateral plantar nerve. The sural nerve can be compressed at any point along its course and symptoms can be expected from branches originating distal to the affected site. Common anatomic sites of sural nerve compression are the lateral aspect of the heel or foot, often caused by trauma. Compression also can be caused by a thickened fibrous arch of superficial sural aponeurosis at the junction of the tendo Achilles and the gastrocnemius. Compression occurs at the edges of the nonextensible tunnel formed by the folds of the posterior aponeurosis.[10]

### Clinical presentation

The first published description of the clinic sequelae of sural nerve entrapment neuropathy was published in 1974.[11] These patients commonly will recall injury to the affected extremity, most often frequent or recurrent "ankle sprains." Other conditions, such as fractures of the calcaneus or fifth metatarsal, chronic Achilles tendonitis, or a space-occupying lesion, such as a ganglion, have been associated with sural nerve entrapments.[12] Less common conditions that have been reported in the literature as causative for sural nerve entrapment include a sural nerve course that pierces the gastrocnemius[7,13] (often made worse after an injury to the gastrocnemius[14]), as well as entrapment from the short saphenous vein.[15] Patients will often complain of chronic burning, numbness, or aching about the posterolateral aspect of the leg, which frequently becomes worse at night and with physical exertion. The pain is sometimes described as "radiating" or "tingling" and may be referred either proximally into the gastrocnemius or distally into the foot, usually along the lateral border of the foot and/or involving the lateral toes. Clinical examination is often otherwise unremarkable, as reflex and motor examinations are not usually affected. Often there is mild to moderate tenderness to palpation posterior and lateral to the myotendinous junction of the Achilles tendon, which represents the location of the fibrous arcade and the most common site of sural nerve entrapment. Reproduction of localized or neuritic distal pain with percussion testing along the course of the nerve can be helpful, although some studies have noted that Tinel will be negative in most of these patients.[13] Furthermore, provocative testing through placing the nerve on stretch, in a dorsiflexed, inverted position, may reproduce symptoms.[12]

Iatrogenic etiologies of sural nerve injury include tendo Achilles surgery, particularly with approaches on the lateral side of the tendon, which may injure either the branch along the lateral side or the main nerve, either by direct injury or indirectly by induration of the wound. A posterolateral ankle arthroscopy portal may put the nerve in danger, as well as surgical repair of a calcaneal fracture. Lateral ankle ligament reconstruction may also put the nerve in jeopardy, as well as fixation of a fifth metatarsal fracture.

### Diagnostic studies

The diagnosis of nerve entrapment syndromes is primarily based on history, symptomology, and physical diagnosis. Plain radiographs are an excellent first-line study, as this condition can result following traumatic injury to the foot or ankle and the potential for robust fracture callous impinging on the course of the nerve should be considered. Stress views should be considered if a history of repetitive trauma to the ankle or a physical examination finding of increased laxity is present. Other modalities such as ultrasound allow for detailed measurements of nerve caliber and can often assist in localizing the site of nerve compression. MRI is often helpful for detailing fine nervous structures and identifying areas of edema and compression through the course of the nerve. MRI is also important in the characterization of space-occupying lesions that may impinge on the nerve. Although CT provides less detail in terms of soft tissue contents, it can be a useful adjunct when physical examination suggests an osseous structure is contributing to impingement or compression of a peripheral nerve or neurovascular bundle.[16] Although there have been improvements in the ability to diagnose this condition through electrodiagnostic studies, the anatomic variation of this nerve in the foot and ankle presents ongoing challenges to interpret even the most careful study. This can limit the usefulness of the study, although it may be helpful in certain situations to rule out other disorders (such as a polyneuropathy).

### Treatment

Successful treatment of sural nerve–related entrapment depends on localization of the site of entrapment. In-office local anesthetic injections at suspected areas of entrapment can assist with diagnosis and short-term treatment if relief of symptoms is achieved.[17] Other general medical conditions, such as peripheral edema or instability of the ankle, should first be addressed. Conservative measures should be targeted at the suspected underlying mechanism. Other modalities for treatment include anti-inflammatory medication, shoe wear modification, and/or inserts to reduce foot contact pressures.[17]

Definitive treatment for this condition is surgical and involves localization and release of the cause of the nerve entrapment. Various investigators have suggested that local exploration and decompression should be reserved for patients with a well-localized and consistent area of pain to repetitive testing who have failed nonoperative measurements.[12,18] Preoperative imaging studies can assist in determining other lesions underlying nerve pain that may be amenable to surgical resection, such as fracture callus or ganglion. Nerve injury resulting in neuroma should either be resected or transposed to an area less vulnerable to injury.[12] High resection of the nerve may be indicated, allowing the nerve to retract between the gastrocnemius heads. However, it is important to remember the peroneal communicating branch and to do the resection distally instead or as well. I often resect just proximal to the ankle, allowing the nerve to retract into more padded tissues, or bury the nerve under the gastrocnemius fascia or into the soleus.

### Saphenous Nerve Entrapment

Saphenous nerve entrapment is a rare condition that has a variety of clinical presentations.

### Anatomy

The saphenous nerve is the longest and terminal branch of the femoral nerve and primarily functions to provide sensory function to the medial aspect of the distal foot. The fibers of the saphenous nerve originate from L3 and L4 and traverse a long distance through the leg, leading to multiple potential sites for entrapment throughout the leg.[19] The saphenous nerve originates distal to the inguinal ligament, descends through the femoral triangle, and joins the femoral artery and vein as it passes through the adductor canal. The nerve then becomes superficial as it passes between the sartorious and the gracilis, piercing the fascia lata. It continues distally on the medial side of the leg, traveling with the greater saphenous vein. The infrapatellar branch of the nerve exits the adductor canal and supplies the anteromedial aspect of the knee. Studies have shown that a large part of the anatomic variability in the saphenous nerve relates to the point at which the infrapatellar branch exits the adductor canal to become a subcutaneous structure.[20] Interestingly, when variable anatomy is observed in this nerve, it is usually identical bilaterally.[21] This branch supplies the skin over the medial side and front of the knee and patellar ligament. Next, the nerve courses distally along the tibial side of the leg, now accompanied by the great saphenous vein. The saphenous nerve descends along the medial tibial border and divides into 2 branches in the distal aspect of the leg. The medial crural cutaneous branches supply sensation to the skin of the front and medial side of the leg and communicate with cutaneous branches of the femoral nerve. The remainder of the saphenous nerve continuoo diotally and at the level of the ankle lays between the anterior tibial tendon and the medial malleolus, just lateral to the saphenous vein. The nerve supplies the dorsum of the foot, medial malleolus, and skin overlying the first metatarsal head.

The course of the saphenous nerve is long and subject to compression at a number of anatomic sites. As the nerve travels distally toward the foot and ankle, it can also be compressed just distal to the adductor canal as it becomes subcutaneous. The infrapatellar branch of the saphenous nerve is often sacrificed with large longitudinal incisions, such as the midline approach to the knee for total knee replacement. This nerve is often cited in the generation of medial knee pain, particularly in athletes and those with chronic knee pain.[19,22,23] In addition, more distal compression or injury to the nerve can be referred to the knee, with the putative mechanism being through the infrapatellar branch of the saphenous nerve. As the nerve continues distally, it runs superficially down the anteromedial aspect of the leg, lateral to the greater saphenous vein. As the nerve descends, at least 3 major cutaneous branches (middle anterior, middle posterior, and inferior anterior) to the anterior leg are given off. At the level of the ankle, the saphenous nerve continues its course just lateral to the saphenous vein, between the medial malleolus and anterior tibial tendon. The nerve then branches and terminates distally in the foot, supplying the medial and side of the foot to approximately the level of the medial side of the first metatarsophalangeal (MTP) joint. The most frequent iatrogenic injury to the distal nerve is harvest of the greater saphenous vein in the course of coronary artery bypass surgery.

### Clinical presentation
Saphenous nerve entrapment can present in a variety of ways depending primarily on the site of nerve compression. Isolated compression of the infrapatellar branch of the nerve is not uncommon, and should be considered in cases of atypical or refractory knee pain and following trauma to the medial side of the knee. These patients will also notice a worsening of the pain with knee flexion or with use of braces that circumferentially encompass this area of the leg. More distal impingement usually results in pain, numbness, or paresthesia localized to the medial side of the leg or foot.

Physical examination should include examination of both muscle strength and sensation in the distal aspects of the leg and foot. Although the nerve is sensory and muscle wasting is unexpected, it may be seen because of disuse atrophy. Frank or extensive muscle wasting suggests that a more proximal location of nerve entrapment should be investigated. The nerve is palpated about its course from proximal to the medial condyle of the femur, down the medial side of the leg to the foot. Localized tenderness may be observed, and the hallmark of diagnosis is tenderness to palpation along the course of the nerve, often also with a reproducible Tinel sign at the site of entrapment.[19] Relief of pain with injection of a local anesthetic suggests localization of a more precise site of entrapment. Paresthesia or dysesthesia may also be noted on the medial side of the leg or medial foot, typically proximal to the first MTP joint.

### Diagnostic studies
When saphenous nerve entrapment is suspected, radiographs provide an excellent first-line examination. Radiographs should be routinely obtained in cases of trauma to rule out fracture and possible resulting bony impingement on the nerve. Advanced diagnostic studies such as MRI or CT are not routinely indicated but can be considered to more clearly elucidate bony structures surrounding the course of the nerve (CT) or for preoperative planning and more precise localization of impingement in cases refractory to conservative measures. Nerve conduction studies are available to assess the main branch of the saphenous nerve or the terminal branches.[24] However, routine testing may not yield useful results in patients with significant subcutaneous adipose tissue or swelling of the extremity.[25] When used, side-to-side comparisons should be performed and any positive results should be correlated with the patient's clinical complaints. Electromyography (EMG) for suspected saphenous nerve impingement should include testing of the adductor longus and quadriceps muscles. In almost all cases, one expects EMG to be negative. In the event it shows findings in either of these 2 proximal muscle groups, radiculopathy should be considered.

### Treatment
Initial treatment for saphenous nerve impingement pain is conservative therapy. Any underlying extrinsic factors, such as the presence of a tumor or fracture impinging on the course of the nerve, should be ruled out. Activity modification and physical therapy, with a focus on strengthening and usage of proper body mechanics, may help to alleviate pain in some patients. Nonsteroidal medications, topical analgesics,

and systemic nerve modulators (such as gabapentin or tricyclic antidepressants) are generally recommended.[19] Local injections of anesthetic with or without steroid may provide relief in some cases. Injections should be focused on the area of most intense pain. Patients with intractable pain who fail conservative measures, therapy, and activity modification should be considered for surgery.[26]

In general, conservative measures should be exhausted before initiating surgical management.[26] Surgical options include decompression, neurectomy, and neurolysis. Decompression and/or neurolysis are generally favored given that neurectomy results in permanent sensory deficits.[19] Studies on decompression and neurolysis have generally demonstrated a reduction or elimination of pain in 60% to 80% of cases, although follow-up in most studies was limited and a large number of patients went on to require neurectomy.[27–29]

## Common Peroneal Nerve Entrapment

### Anatomy

The common peroneal nerve arises at about the level of the mid-thigh as a branch of the sciatic nerve. Its fibers originate from the L4, L5, S1, and S2 nerve roots. The nerve travels in the posterior compartment of the thigh and provides innervation for the short head of the biceps femoris. The nerve crosses posterior to the lateral head of the gastrocnemius as it descends obliquely on the lateral side of the popliteal fossa, close to the medial margin of the biceps femoris. It becomes subcutaneous posterior to the fibular head, lying between the tendon of the biceps femoris and the lateral head of the gastrocnemius before passing distally around the fibular neck between the fibula and the peroneus longus (**Fig. 1**). It then divides, forming the deep and superficial peroneal nerves. It is important to note, however, that cadaveric studies have shown significant anatomic variability in this region, with one cadaveric study indicating that the site of branching occurs up to 5 cm proximal to the knee joint in some cases.[30]

### Clinical presentation

Peroneal nerve injury occurs secondary to a large number of etiologies that can affect the nerve at any point along its course. The clinical presentation is highly dependent on the site of compression. The most frequent point of injury of this nerve occurs in the vicinity of the fibular head secondary to a direct trauma.[31] There are a large number of other causes for peroneal nerve dysfunction, which are generally divided into 2 categories: a result of external factors (such as habitual leg crossing,[32] pressure from prolonged positioning as can occur in debilitated patients or those undergoing surgery, pressure from prolonged squatting, tall boots, casts or braces, or tight shoe laces) or secondary to internal factors (fractures resulting in tension on the nerve, neoplasm, vascular abnormality, exercise-induced compartment syndrome, lacerations of the nerve, or postsurgical entrapment from sutures or hardware). Other less common causes that have been reported in the literature include compression secondary to a lipoma,[33] tibiofibular ganglion cysts,[34] popliteal venous aneurysms,[35] proximal posterior tibial osseous tumors, secondary to severe burn injury,[36] and after total knee replacements.[37]

Clinically, patients with common peroneal nerve injuries present with a variety of complaints, dependent mostly upon the location of the lesion. More proximal lesions commonly present with the patient complaining of difficult or uncoordinated gait secondary to loss of strength or ability to dorsiflex the ankle. Pain is not a constant in common peroneal nerve injuries and is often dependent upon the injury (ie, traumatic wounds will have associated pain, chronic entrapment or compression may present with or without pain and with or without distal areas of anesthesia). Loss of

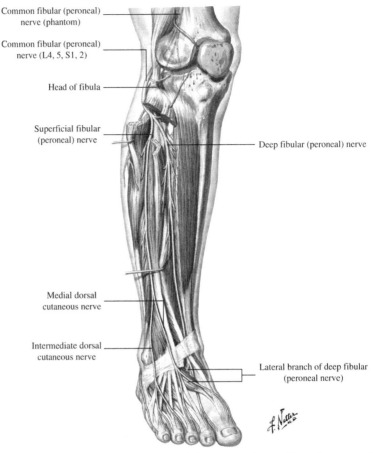

Common fibular (peroneal) nerve (phantom)

Common fibular (peroneal) nerve (L4, 5, S1, 2)

Head of fibula

Superficial fibular (peroneal) nerve

Deep fibular (peroneal) nerve

Medial dorsal cutaneous nerve

Intermediate dorsal cutaneous nerve

Lateral branch of deep fibular (peroneal nerve)

**Fig. 1.** Illustration of a superficial dissection of the anterior leg and foot demonstrating the course and terminal branches for the common, superficial, and deep peroneal nerves. The common peroneal nerve wraps around the head of the fibula before dividing into the deep and superficial peroneal nerves. The superficial peroneal nerve is important for its subcutaneous location over the fibula, classically described as 10 to 12 cm above the tip of the lateral malleolus. This nerve can sustain iatrogenic injuries as a result of any incision using a lateral approach to the ankle. When using this approach to the fibula, the nerve should ideally be identified and protected. (Netter illustration from www.netterimages. com. © Elsevier Inc. All rights reserved.)

sensation can be seen in varying distributions depending on both the patient's individual anatomic variations as well as the precise location of the lesion. A steppage gait is commonly observed with increased flexion of the hip and knee to compensate for the loss of ankle dorsiflexion strength.

Physical examination should focus first on identifying any obvious injuries in the distribution of the nerve. For example, a fracture of the fibular head that lacerates or compresses the peroneal nerve can result in foot drop and complete anesthesia to the dorsum of the foot. The limited superficial course of the nerve makes palpation difficult, but response to Tinel test can be assessed at the fibular neck. Positive Tinel sign commonly results in tingling along the course and in the distal distribution of the peroneal nerve. Tinel sign is an excellent adjunct to diagnosis, as a study demonstrated that 97% of patients with this condition had a positive Tinel.[38] Gait should be assessed as noted previously with particular concern for a foot-drop and/or steppage-type gait patterns resulting from loss of ankle dorsiflexion strength. Often a "slapping" sound will be produced as these patients walk owing to their inability to control descent of the foot to the floor. In much the same manner, muscle strength testing focusing on ankle dorsiflexion and extensor digitorum brevis (EDB) strength should be assessed. Of note, patients can present with relative sparing of the ankle everters. Thus, examination for dorsiflexion strength should be conducted with the foot in inversion to properly isolate the tibialis anterior.[39] Sensation should be carefully assessed, as these findings can assist with diagnosis.

### Diagnostic studies
First-line studies for assessing common peroneal injury should be plain radiographs, given the proximity of the nerve to the fibular neck and potential for impingement secondary to trauma, tumor, or bony exostosis. CT scans play an adjunct role in the assessment of nerve lesions from underlying bony abnormalities, particularly (although not limited to) fractures. Similarly, MRI scans play a limited role in assisting to elucidate the position and composition of a soft tissue mass that is suspected to lie in the course of the common peroneal nerve. Electrodiagnostic studies are often useful in common peroneal nerve dysfunctions in differentiating the location of a lesion. This test can assist in determining the relative location of the lesion, as well as detailing the possibility of more proximal involvement (such as the L5 nerve root). Clinically, the determination of the lesion as being proximal or distal to the knee hinges on evaluation of the short head of the biceps, a difficult determination to make on physical examination.[39] Both sensory and motor conduction studies are necessary for a full diagnosis. A superficial peroneal sensory nerve action potential (SNAP) is tested, and abnormality (typically in the form of loss of amplitude) implies some axonal loss affecting the nerve distal to the dorsal root ganglion. However, a SNAP alone does not allow for localization of the lesion. Motor conduction studies should also be con-ducted with the active electrode placed in the EDB muscle. Stimulation is then provided both proximal and distal to the fibular head, which allows for assessment of the nerve across the fibular neck, a common site of injury. Conduction velocity of less than 40 m/s is generally considered abnormal and the contralateral side should be assessed as well for comparison. Needle EMG can also be useful in determining the involvement (or lack of involvement) of either the superficial or deep branches of the peroneal. In conjunction with EMG of the short head of the biceps femoris, the proximal extent of the lesion can be defined. Testing muscles innervated by the tibial nerve can also assist in determining potential involvement of the L5 nerve roots (abnor-malities expected in muscles innervated by both tibial and peroneal nerves if the nerve root is involved).[39]

### Treatment
Treatment of common peroneal nerve injuries is largely dependent upon determination of the underlying cause; however, a recent retrospective review of 146 cases deter-mined that fully 38% of cases were felt to be "idiopathic" in nature.[40] Nonoperative treatment of peroneal nerve injuries is generally indicated for a period of approximately 3 to 4 months, as there have been reports in the literature of spontaneous resolution of symptoms, particularly when some degree of nerve function remains. Nonsurgical options that reliably lead to resolution of symptoms are generally more limited for common peroneal involvement than for other compression neuropathies. Anti-inflammatory medications are a reasonable first-line treatment in cases where

inflammation or swelling may be causing entrapment. Corticosteroid injection may also reduce swelling, and when combined with local anesthetic can assist in localizing the lesion. Tricyclic antidepressants have been commonly used for nerve-related pain along with medications such as gabapentin, carbamazepine, and tramadol. Recent studies have suggested that the tricyclic medications should be used first, as they had the most favorable number needed to treat (NNT) for pain relief versus other types of nerve pain–modulating agents.[41]

Nonoperative, symptomatic treatment of muscular symptoms such as foot drop can be accomplished with the use of orthotics such as an ankle-foot orthosis (AFO). Biomechanical correction of foot position through the use of insoles or wedges may also provide some relief.[39]

Surgical treatment is generally indicated when conservative measures have failed to provide adequate relief or restoration of function. In some cases, such as intraneuronal ganglion cysts, early surgical treatment may be more beneficial than an attempt at conservative management.[42] Fabre and colleagues[38] suggested surgical intervention via open decompression of the peroneal nerve after 3 to 4 months without resolution of symptoms. Conditions causing severe paresis or significant muscle atrophy should also be considered for early surgical intervention.

Aside from addressing an underlying diagnosis, surgical decompression is the most common method of restoring function in common peroneal nerve entrapment. Fabre and colleagues[38] describe an open release of the common peroneal nerve, isolated posteromedial to the biceps femoris. The nerve is followed distally to the bifurcation, and the deep distal band of the fibrous arch is released. The lateral septum is then separated and the superficial portion of the arch is exposed and completely released until the nerve is free of impingement. Using this technique, Fabre and colleagues[38] reported symptomatic improvement in all 7 patients with postural symptoms (ie, related to a particular position that placed stress or stretch on the nerve) and in 79% (42 of 53 patients) of patients with idiopathic or pain from unknown causes. They noted a higher incidence of failure in patients who had symptoms of long duration before surgery. They also cite failures in causes of polyneuropathy (such as alcohol related) to the point that they now consider polyneuropathy a contraindication to surgery and do not typically recommend surgery for patients with sensory symptoms lasting longer than 24 months. Other studies have demonstrated similar findings, with improvement observed in 84% of patients with preoperative pain and in 83% of patients with preoperative motor weakness, compared with only 49% of patients with sensory disturbances noted preoperatively.[43] The available evidence suggests a benefit to early decompression at 3 to 4 months after the onset of symptoms. If full release of the superficial and deep aspects of the fibrous arch is achieved, the expected outcome is quite good for patients with primarily motor complaints and without polyneuropathy.

### Superficial Peroneal Nerve Entrapment

Entrapment or impingement of the superficial peroneal nerve (SPN) is referred to as mononeuralgia of the peroneal nerve and was first described by Henry in 1945.[44] It is a relatively rare condition, with a 1997 study of nearly 500 patients with chronic leg pain showing only 3.5% attributable to entrapment of the SPN.[45]

### Anatomy

The SPN remains lateral following the bifurcation from the common peroneal nerve and supplies motor innervation in the lateral compartment of the leg. The nerve passes deep to the peroneus longus, traveling between this muscle and the fibula in the lateral compartment. It becomes more superficial as it courses distally between the peroneus longus and the brevis before piercing the fascia through the crural tunnel, at a level classically noted to be approximately 10 to 12 cm proximal to the tip of the lateral malleolus (see **Fig. 1**). Because of the surgical relevance of this nerve in ankle fractures, the course and significant amount of variation present in this nerve has been the subject of numerous studies over the years.[26,46] These studies demonstrated that not only does the distal-proximal location at which the nerve pierces the lateral compartment fascia vary, but in some cases the nerve does not pierce the lateral compartment fascia at all. Rather, in 14% of cadaveric limbs the investigators saw the nerve passing into and subsequently exiting from the anterior compartment fascia, whereas in another 12% the nerve bifurcated proximally, with one limb exiting the lateral fascia and the other exiting the anterior fascia.[46] As the nerve continues distally, it typically divides again into the intermediate and medial dorsal cutaneous nerve about 6 to 7 cm distal to the tip of the fibula. Distally, the nerve branches to form the medial and intermediate cutaneous nerves to the foot. The medial branch travels lateral to the extensor hallucis longus (EHL) tendon, supplying sensation to the medial dorsum of the foot, including the great, second, and often the third toe. The intermediate branch passes medial to the lateral malleolus and can often be visualized as it becomes superficial passing over the sinus tarsi. It then continues on the dorsum of the foot, typically providing sensory innervation to the lateral third, fourth, and fifth toes.

### Clinical presentation

Localized trauma to the nerve is the most common underlying cause of entrapment. The classically described superficial peroneal nerve injury occurs in the setting of repeated ankle sprains (particularly ankle inversion injuries), thought to be a result of the traction placed on the nerve.[47] Some patients may report the pain as similar to an ankle sprain that fails to resolve.[48] Positions that consistently place the nerve on stretch, such as prolonged kneeling or squatting, may predispose to the development of superficial peroneal nerve symptomatology. The injury has been described in dancers and other athletes with lateral ligament deficiency or functional ankle instability where the nerve is repeatedly subjected to stretching forces. These individuals also are at increased risk secondary to their often hypertrophic peroneal musculature that can result in entrapment of the nerve in its short fibrous tunnel as it pierces the fascia.[49] Iatrogenic injuries can also occur as a consequence of procedures approaching the ankle anteriorly, including ankle arthroscopy. Ankle arthroscopy studies have demonstrated a 2.0% to 2.5% incidence of injury to branches of the superficial peroneal nerve, either as a result of direct trauma from portal placement or secondary to stretch injury owing to traction required for the procedure.[50,51] Exertional compartment syndrome[52] and anatomic variability, including fascial defects can also result in impingement. The investigators have also noted sequelae of iatrogenic injury of the superficial peroneal nerve related to the lateral approach to the fibula for ankle fractures. Typically, these injuries occur on revision procedures or ankle hardware removal after a fracture. It is likely that the aberrant postsurgical anatomy and scar tissue make visualization difficult and place the nerve at increased risk of injury. Surgery involving the dorsal tarsus for midtarsal and tarsometatarsal arthritis are further opportunities for nerve injury.

As with other nerve pathologies, the site of nerve compression greatly influences the clinical presentation. Diagnosis is also complicated by the presence of coexisting pathologies that can cause, enhance, or mimic nerve entrapment, such as the presence of a neoplasm or exertional compartment syndrome. Patients with pathology occurring proximal to the innervation of the lateral compartment can present with muscular symptoms, particularly reduced ankle eversion and plantarflexion owing to loss of innervation to the peroneus longus and brevis. Impingement distal to these points most often results in sensory complaints.

Clinical presentation is likewise variable for these patients. Classically, pain is localized to the mid to distal third of the leg, often concentrating on the anterior aspect of the leg with radiation to the dorsal aspect of the foot. Night pain and pain at rest are rare, although symptoms are commonly aggravated by activity. Examination of the foot reveals no specific motor weakness, and approximately two-thirds will have no sensory loss in the foot.[53] The course of the nerve should be palpated, and often will reveal sensitivity to palpation most commonly at the site where the nerve pierces the crural fascia.

Styf[44] proposed 3 provocative maneuvers designed to place the nerve on stretch that can be used to assist in diagnosis. First, one should palpate and hold pressure over the site of entrapment while the patient actively dorsiflexes and everts the foot against resistance. Second, the examiner should passively plantarflex and invert the ankle. Third, the examiner should percuss over the course of the nerve while passively maintaining stretch with ankle inversion. Positive results are defined as a finding of pain/paresthesia in 2 of these 3 provocative maneuvers. More recently, the fourth toe flexion sign has been described as a method to accentuate the subcutaneous course of the cutaneous branches of the SPN. The investigators found that injection of anesthetic in this area resulted in delineation of the distribution of the SPN in 86% of patients, which could assist in the diagnosis of dorsal foot pain as originating from the SPN.[54]

### Diagnostic studies
Standard workup should include radiographs to rule out bony impingement secondary to injury or prior fracture. There are case reports of SPN entrapment secondary to abundant fracture callous following fibular fractures.[55] Furthermore, the presence of exostoses or osteochondromas may result in impingement anywhere along the course of the nerve. CT scan may provide more detailed information if bony involvement in the impingement is suspected following plain radiography. MRI can be useful to delineate soft tissue involvements, and may be particularly useful in examining the passage of the nerve through the crural fascia or in cases where soft tissue lesions are felt to be compressing the nerve. Ultrasound can be helpful to identify a cystic mass impinging on the nerve.

Nerve conduction studies in the superficial peroneal nerve are performed in a standardized fashion and results are able to be obtained in nearly 98% of patients.[56] Although most investigators concede that nerve conduction studies should be regarded as adjuncts for diagnosis and reserved for situations where the diagnosis is in question, studies have shown reproducible and consistent changes to conduction velocity in the SPN in cases of impingement. Styf and Morberg[45] found a nonsignificant decrease in conduction velocity from 49 m/s in unaffected nerves, to 28 m/s on average on the affected side. Other studies have shown increased latencies and attenuation of action potentials. It is important to remember that normal nerve conduction studies do not rule out SPN involvement and thus must be viewed as only a tool to assist in diagnosis.

Localized injection of anesthetic at the site of maximal tenderness can serve as both a diagnostic as well as a therapeutic intervention. Relief of symptoms is generally considered to indicate the site of involvement, which can also assist with preoperative planning if surgical intervention is eventually required.

*Treatment*

In general, the superficial nerve is felt to respond less well to conservative measures than the deep peroneal nerve.[57] Once SPN entrapment is diagnosed, conservative measures should generally be exhausted before progressing to surgical decompression. Lateral shoe wedges may help to reduce varus stress on the ankle and thus the nerve. Use of nonsteroidal anti-inflammatory drugs (NSAIDs) and relative rest can be attempted, and patients should be told to avoid shoes or boots that constrict the distal ankle and foot. Physical therapy focusing on ankle strengthening and range of motion can be useful, particularly when lateral ligament deficiency or functional ankle instability is present. Cortisone injections, with or without the addition of local anesthetics, at the site of nerve entrapment, may also provide relief. The use of Botox under ultrasound guidance has been described in a case report to treat SPN entrapment secondary to muscle herniation through a fascial defect of the lateral compartment and may represent a future avenue of care for a subgroup of these patients.[58]

When these measures have failed, surgical intervention is warranted. Typically, surgical intervention is described as release of the SPN from the surrounding fascia at the point where it exits the crural fascia. Past wisdom was that the fascia of lateral compartment should be completely released in cases of superficial nerve entrapment. Although this advice is still valid when these symptoms occur concurrently with exertional compartment syndromes, more recent studies support a more limited dissection. Before surgery the nerve should be percussed to determine the site of compression and marked. Surgical dissection should identify the peroneal tunnel, a fibrous structure found to vary in length from 3 to 11 cm, which is the common site of compression. One study advocates complete opening of the peroneal tunnel close to the anterior intermuscular septum. In this small series, 80% of patients reported relief of symptoms.[45] Other more recent studies also support a more limited 3- to 5-cm incision centered approximately 5 to 8 cm above the lateral malleolus.[59] More research on long-term outcomes is required for more specific recommendations, but the available evidence supports surgical decompression of either the peroneal tunnel or of both the lateral compartment and the peroneal tunnel in cases that occur in conjunction with an exertional compartment syndrome. When the injury follows a lower-extremity hardware removal and results in a neuroma in continuity, the investigators have had positive anecdotal results with neurectomy and subsequent burying of nerve ends in local muscle.

## Deep Peroneal Nerve Entrapment (Anterior Tarsal Tunnel Syndrome)

*Anatomy*

After branching from the common peroneal nerve, the deep peroneal nerve courses anteriorly around the fibular neck and enters the anterior compartment between peroneus longus and the fibular neck. It courses distally on the surface of the fibula for 3 to 4 cm, eventually piercing the intramuscular septum between the lateral and anterior compartments. This location represents a potential site of entrapment. In the proximal third of the leg the nerve lies between tibialis anterior and extensor digitorum communis (EDC). It courses distally in tandem with the anterior tibial artery, laying just anterior to the interosseous membrane and supplies motor innervation to the tibialis anterior, EDC, EHL, and peroneus tertius (see **Fig. 1**). At approximately 5 cm proximal to the ankle joint, it lies between the EDC and EHL as it passes underneath the superficial extensor retinaculum. As it continues distally, the nerve branches at a position typically 1 cm proximal to the ankle joint. One mixed branch courses laterally to innervate the EDB and provide sensation to the lateral tarsal joints. The other branch, composed of only sensory fibers, runs distally with the dorsalis pedis artery between the EDC and

EHB tendons and ultimately provides cutaneous innervation in the first dorsal web space. This branch passes underneath the 2 bands of the Y-shaped inferior extensor retinaculum (**Fig. 2**). This is the site of the "anterior tarsal tunnel," an approximately 1.5-cm confined space formed superficially by the inferior extensor retinaculum, deep by the capsule of the talonavicular joint, laterally by the lateral malleolus and medially by the medial malleolus.[60] Through this space courses the dorsalis pedis artery and vein, the deep peroneal nerve, and tendons of the EHL, EDC, tibialis anterior, and peroneus tertius.[61]

### Clinical presentation
A variety of etiologies can lead to clinical symptoms of deep peroneal nerve entrapment. Any space-occupying lesion (neoplasm, osteophytes, fracture, muscle hypertrophy, and so forth) that impinges on the nerve can result in symptomatology. Extrinsic forces such as recurrent ankle sprains, chronic ligamentous laxity, or tight shoe wear (classically in narrow shoes, ski boots) can also cause pain.[53] Rare causes described throughout the literature also include runners who attach a key under the

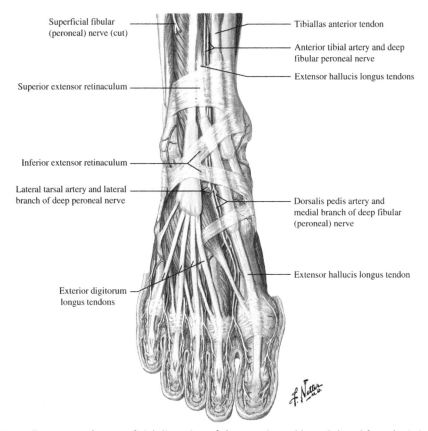

**Fig. 2.** Illustration of a superficial dissection of the anterior ankle and dorsal foot depicting the superior extensor retinaculum above the ankle and the Y-shaped inferior extensor retinaculum, the site of compression in anterior tarsal tunnel syndrome affecting the deep peroneal nerve. Along with the nerve, the dorsalis pedis artery and vein, the deep peroneal nerve, and tendons of the EHL, EDL, tibialis anterior, and peroneus tertius pass through this space. (Netter illustration from www.netterimages.com. © Elsevier Inc. All rights reserved.)

tongue of their shoes and persons doing repetitive exercises like sit-ups with the dorsum of the foot anchored under a solid bar.

Anterior tarsal tunnel syndrome classically presents with vague sensations of pain or burning sensations over the dorsum of the foot. Some also will report paresthesia in the first dorsal webspace. These symptoms can often be exacerbated with plantar-flexion of the foot, a position that places stretch on the nerve and compresses the contents of the anterior tarsal tunnel against the dorsal aspect of the talonavicular joint. The pain is commonly described as increasing with activity and resolves with rest, although night pain also has been commonly described with anterior tarsal tunnel syndrome more so than other types of nerve entrapment.[62] These symptoms can also be seen in patients with exertional anterolateral compartment syndrome, and this condition can be an underlying cause of nerve compression exacerbated with activity.[63] Patients may be able to connect the pain with specific shoe wear or a specific activity, which can assist in making the diagnosis. Lesions or entrapment occurring proximal to the motor branch of the nerve may also result in EDB weakness, which occasionally can be detectable on examination, most commonly as a subtle decrease in extension strength of the toes. Some investigators also suggest direct palpation of the EDB with the patient in active dorsiflexion as a more precise method of determining compromise to innervation of the nerve.

Clinical examination of the patient with suspected anterior tarsal tunnel syndrome or dorsal foot pain should begin with palpation of the deep peroneal nerve along its entire course. The proximal course of the nerve near the fibular neck should also be examined as tenderness is often elicited to percussion (Tinel sign) at the site of entrapment or along the course of the nerve distally. Forceful plantarflexion and inversion of the ankle places the nerve on stretch and decreases the available space in the anterior tarsal tunnel resulting in compression of the nerve against the floor of the tunnel. This maneuver may elicit symptoms over the dorsum of the foot, which can assist in diagnosis.[64] A careful motor examination is also indicated as mentioned before. The subtle weakness caused by decreased or loss of innervation to the EDB is often difficult to detect. Palpating the EDB while the patient actively dorsiflexes the great toes may detect loss of the contribution of this muscle.

### Diagnostic studies

Plain radiographs, often of limited value in other suspected nerve entrapments, play a prominent role when anterior tarsal tunnel syndrome is suspected. Often a lateral view of the foot will demonstrate the presence of dorsal osteophytes, particularly at the talonavicular joint. Radiographs may also reveal fractures, bone fragments, or soft tissue swelling near the course of the nerve. CT scans would appear to have a more limited role, but could be of assistance in better elucidating the bony alignment of a fracture with corresponding nerve involvement. Similarly, MRI has a limited role in diagnosis of the condition, but may be very important if the underlying etiology is felt to be secondary to impingement from an adjacent mass. In these cases, MRI can help identify the mass and can assist in preoperative planning to address nerve decompression and/or excision of the mass.

Electrodiagnostic studies may be useful in diagnosing deep peroneal nerve entrapment, particularly in helping to determine whether there is involvement of the EDB, which suggests a lesion proximal to the inferior retinaculum.[12] Findings suggestive of a nerve-related abnormality on electrodiagnostic study include increased latency and reduced motor recruitment of the EDB; however, these studies are technically difficult to perform. Furthermore, a past study demonstrated abnormal signals (typically defined as latency of conduction greater than 5 ms) in approximately 76% of asymptomatic individuals and decreased EDB motor recruitment in 38% of asymptomatic individuals.[65] Anatomic variations of the nerve also allow the possibility that patients with a normal EDB response on testing may still have an underlying deep peroneal lesion.

Exercise testing, with or without measurement of compartment pressures, may be useful in patients where an exercise-induced compartment syndrome is suspected as the etiologic agent in nerve compression.

With the recent increase in total ankle arthroplasty, the approach between the extensor hallucis longus and the anterior tibial tendons is used frequently. With the neurovascular bundle including the deep perineal nerve under the extensor hallucis, closure of the deep layer under the tendons puts the deep perineal nerve at risk and increasing numbers of deep perineal nerve injuries are being observed.

### Treatment

Nonoperative management can often be helpful in the treatment of deep peroneal nerve entrapment. The primary goal is identification and treatment of the underlying condition resulting in compression of the nerve. Attention should be focused on reducing pressure on the dorsal foot, either through the use of accommodative, nonrestrictive shoe wear or avoidance of shoes that fit or lace tightly over the dorsum of the foot.[64] Orthotics aimed at improving biomechanical alignment of the foot (such as correcting flatfoot or cavus alignment) are reasonable to try in appropriate patients. Physical therapy can be particularly useful when chronic ankle instability occurs in conjunction with nerve symptoms. NSAIDs or other anti-inflammatory pain medication should also be used. Finally, localized injection of corticosteroid and anesthetic may also be attempted in cases where localization of the lesion is possible. Treatments such as these should be exhausted before progressing to surgical management.

Surgical options for deep peroneal nerve entrapment vary depending on the underlying etiology. Symptoms and clinical findings consistent with compression at the anterior tarsal tunnel often respond to decompression of the anterior tarsal tunnel. A straight vertical or S-shaped incision can be used, beginning at the base of the first and second metatarsals and extending proximally to the ankle joint. As the incision is carried deep, branches of the superficial peroneal nerve should be visualized and preserved. The extensor retinaculum is released to the extent necessary to free up the nerve. Past studies suggest that it is desirable to preserve a portion of the extensor retinaculum if possible.[12] Osteophytes or similar structures present on the dorsal edge of the talonavicular joint should be visualized and removed. A 1990 study by Dellon[66] examining results after surgical release of the deep peroneal nerve noted good or excellent results in 80% of patients at 2 years, and no improvement in 20%. In some cases, the EHB may be notably hypertrophied and causing compression of the nerve with thick fibrous bands. Resection of a segment of EHB tendon with transfer to the EHL, along with excision or dorsal osteophytes and release of deep fascia in the midfoot, lead to very good to excellent pain relief in most patients at greater than 6 month follow-up.[67] Simple closure and soft dressings are recommended postoperatively and activity can gradually be resumed over the ensuing 4 to 6 weeks.

### SUMMARY

This article has reviewed a number of common nerve entrapments of the lower extremity, focusing on involvement of the sural, saphenous and common, deep, and superficial peroneal nerves. A working knowledge of the anatomy and the potential variations present in these nerves will greatly assist in diagnosis of this heterogeneous group of conditions. Combining this with appropriate history, physical examination, and judicious use of imaging modalities and/or electrodiagnostic studies will help to elucidate the underlying cause of nerve-related pain.

It is important to remember that nerve compressions often occur in the setting of a systemic condition. Addressing the underlying systemic issues while simultaneously instituting conservative measures to address the nerve compression is a prudent early course of action. Appropriate diagnostic studies, including physical examination, injections, and the use of imaging and/or electrodiagnostic studies will allow further delineation of the exact location of compression. When systemic conditions have been optimized, conservative measures have failed, and a relatively precise location of entrapment has been elucidated, surgical management can be considered. In these cases surgical intervention—most often decompression of the surrounding structures—can be successful in relieving pain and restoring function.

## REFERENCES

1. Gelberman RH, Eaton R, Urbaniak JR. Peripheral nerve compression. J Bone Joint Surg 1993;75:1854–78.
2. Dahlin LB, McLean WG. Effects of graded experimental compression on slow and fast axonal transport in rabbit vagus nerve. J Neurol Sci 1986;72:19–30.
3. Dahlin LB, Shyu BC, Danielsen N, et al. Effects of nerve compression or ischaemia on conduction properties of myelinated and non-myelinated nerve fibres. Acta Physiol Scand 1989;136:97–105.
4. Braidwood AS. Superficial radial neuropathy. J Bone Joint Surg 1975;57:380–3.
5. Rempel D, Dahlin L, Lundborg G, et al. Pathophysiology of nerve compression syndromes: response of peripheral nerves to loading. J Bone Joint Surg 1999; 81:1600–10.
6. Lundborg G, Dahlin LB. Anatomy, function, and pathophysiology of peripheral nerves and nerve compression. Hand Clin 1996;12:185–93.
7. George BM, Nayak S. Sural nerve entrapment in gastrocnemius muscle—a case report. Neuroanatomy 2007;6:41–2.
8. Ortiguela ME, Wood MB, Cahill DR. Anatomy of the sural nerve complex. J Hand Surg Am 1987;12:1119–23.
9. Standring S. In: Gray's anatomy: the anatomical basis of clinical practice. Philadelphia: Churchhill Livingstone; 2004.
10. Husson JL, Mathieu M, Briand B, et al. Syndrome of compression of the sural nerve. Acta Ortop Belg 1989;55:491–7 [in French].
11. Pringle RM, Protheroe K, Mukherjee SK. Entrapment neuropathy of the sural nerve. J Bone Joint Surg Br 1974;56:465–8.
12. Beskin JL. Nerve entrapment syndromes of the foot and ankle. J Am Acad Orthop Surg 1997;5:261–9.
13. Fabre T, Montero C, Gaujard E, et al. Chronic calf pain in athletes due to sural nerve entrapment. A report of 18 cases. Am J Sports Med 2000;28:679–82.
14. Bryan BM, Lutz GE, O'Brien SJ. Sural nerve entrapment after injury to the gastrocnemius: a case report. Arch Phys Med Rehabil 1999;80:604–6.
15. Nayak SB. Sural nerve and short saphenous vein entrapment—a case report. Indian J Plast Surg 2005;38:171–2.
16. Delfaut EM, Demondion X, Bieganski A, et al. Imaging of foot and ankle nerve entrapment syndromes: from well-demonstrated to unfamiliar sites. Radiographics 2003;23:613–23.
17. Bare AA, Haddad SL. Nerve entrapment syndromes. In: Thordarson DB, editor. Foot and ankle. Philadelphia: Lippincott, Williams & Wilkins; 2004. p. 79–97.

18. Myerson M. Management of nerve entrapment syndromes. In: Myerson M, editor. Reconstructive foot and ankle surgery: management of complications. 2nd edition. Philadelphia: Saunders; 2010. Chapter 21.

19. Morganti CM, McFarland EG, Cosgarea AJ. Saphenous neuritis: a poorly understood cause of medial knee pain. J Am Acad Orthop Surg 2002;10:130–7.

20. Dunaway DJ, Steensen RN, Wiand W, et al. The sartorial branch of the saphenous nerve: its anatomy at the joint line of the knee. Arthroscopy 2005;5:547–51.

21. Hunter LY, Louse DS, Ricciardi JR. The saphenous nerve: its course and importance in medial arthrotomy. Am J Sports Med 1979;7:227–30.

22. Key VH. Leg pain in runners. Curr Opin Orthop 2007;18:161–5.

23. Edwards PH, Wright ML, Hartman JF. A practical approach for the differential diagnosis of chronic leg pain in the athlete. Am J Sports Med 2006;33:1241–9.

24. Hemler DE, Ward WK, Karstetter KW, et al. Saphenous nerve entrapment caused by pes anserine bursitis mimicking stress fracture of the tibia. Arch Phys Med Rehabil 1991;72:336–7.

25. Dumitru D. In: Electrodiagnostic medicine. Philadelphia: Hanley and Belfus; 1995.

26. Kalenak A. Saphenous nerve entrapment. Arthroscopy 1996;4:40–5.

27. Worth RM, Kettelkamp DB, Defalque RJ, et al. Saphenous nerve entrapment: a cause of medial knee pain. Am J Sports Med 1984;12:80–1.

28. Kopell HP, Thompson WA. Knee pain due to saphenous-nerve entrapment. N Engl J Med 1960;263:351–3.

29. Luerssen TG, Campbell RL, Defalque RJ, et al. Spontaneous saphenous neuralgia. Neurosurgery 1983;13:238–41.

30. Deutsch A, Wyzkowski RJ, Victoroff BN. Evaluation of the anatomy of the common peroneal nerve. Am J Sports Med 1999;27:10–5.

31. Banerjee T, Koons DD. Superficial peroneal nerve entrapment: report of two cases. J Neurosurg 1981;55:991–2.

32. Kaminsky F. Peroneal palsy by crossing the legs. JAMA 1947;134:206.

33. Hsu YC, Shih YY, Gao HW, et al. Subcutaneous lipoma compressing the common peroneal nerve and causing palsy: sonographic diagnosis. J Clin Ultrasound 2009;38:97–9.

34. Farjoodi P, Johnson TS. Proximal tibiofibular ganglion cyst causing peroneal neuropraxia. Curr Orthop Pract 2010;21:209–12.

35. Jang SH, Lee H, Han SH. Common peroneal nerve compression by a popliteal venous aneurysm. Am J Phys Med Rehabil 2009;88:947–50.

36. Bozkurt A, Grieb G, O'Dey D, et al. Common peroneal nerve compression and heterotopic ossification resulting from severe burn injury. J Bone Joint Surg Am 2010;92:978–83.

37. Idusuyi OB, Morrey BF. Peroneal nerve palsy after total knee arthroplasty. J Bone Joint Surg 1996;78:177–84.

38. Fabre T, Piton C, Andre D, et al. Peroneal nerve entrapment. J Bone Joint Surg 1998;80:47–53.

39. Hollis MH, Lemay DE. Nerve entrapment syndromes of the lower extremity. Emedicine medscape. Updated 7/10/09. Available at: http://emedicine.medscape.com/article/1234809-overview. Accessed January 9, 2010.

40. Piton C, Fabre T, Lasseur E, et al. Common fibular nerve lesions. Etiology and treatment. Apropos of 146 cases with surgical treatment. Rev Chir Orthop Reparatrice Appar Mot 1997;83:515–21 [in French].

41. Sindrup SH, Jensen TS. Pharmacologic treatment of pain in polyneuropathy. Neurology 2000;55:915–20.

42. Lowenstein J, Towers J, Tomaino MM. Intraneural ganglion of the peroneal nerve: importance of timely diagnosis. Am J Orthop 2001;30(11):816–9.

43. Humphreys DB, Novak CB, Mackinnon SE. Patient outcomes after common peroneal nerve decompression. J Neurosurg 2007;107:314–8.

44. Styf J. Entrapment of the superficial peroneal nerve. J Bone Joint Surg Br 1989; 71:131–5.

45. Styf J, Morberg P. The superficial peroneal tunnel syndrome: results of treatment by decompression. J Bone Joint Surg Br 1997;79:801–3.

46. Adkison DP, Bosse MJ, Gaccione DR, et al. Anatomical variations in the course of the superficial peroneal nerve. J Bone Joint Surg Am 1991;73:112–4.

47. O'Neill PJ, Parks BG, Walsh R, et al. Excursion and strain of the superficial peroneal nerve during inversion ankle sprain. J Bone Joint Surg Am 2007;89: 979–86.

48. Kernohan J, Levack B, Wilson NJ. Entrapment of the superficial peroneal nerve: three case reports. J Bone Joint Surg Br 1985;67B:60–1.

49. Kennedy JG, Baxter DE. Nerve disorders in dancers. Clin Sports Med 2008;27: 329–34.

50. Ferkel RD, Heath DD, Guhl JF, et al. Neurological complications of ankle arthroscopy. Arthroscopy 1996;12:200–8.

51. Young BH, Flanigan RM, DiGiovanni BF. Complications of ankle arthroscopy using a contemporary non-invasive distraction technique. J Bone Joint Surg Am, in press.

52. Wilder RP, Magrum EM. Exertional compartment syndrome. Clin Sports Med 2010;29:429–35.

53. Baxter DE. Functional nerve disorders in the athlete's foot, ankle, and leg. Instr Course Lect 1993;42:185–94.

54. Stephens MM, Kelly PM. Fourth toe flexion sign: a new clinical sign for identification of the superficial peroneal nerve. Foot Ankle Int 2000;12:995.

55. Mino D, Hughes EC. Bony entrapment of the superficial peroneal nerve. Clin Orthop Relat Res 1984;185:203–6.

56. Izzo KL, Sridhara CR, Rosenholtz H, et al. Sensory conduction studies of the branches of the superficial peroneal nerve. Arch Phys Med Rehabil 1981;62: 24–7.

57. Pecina M, Krmpotic-Nemanic J, Markiewitz AD. Tunnel syndrome in athletes in tunnel syndromes: peripheral nerve compression syndromes. New York: Taylor & Francis, Inc; 2001. 288–94.

58. Yoo MJ, Kim D, Lee J, et al. Injection of botulinum toxin as a treatment for superficial peroneal nerve ontrapment cause by a muscle hernia: a case report [poster 211]. Arch Phys Med Rehabil 2007;88(9):E70. Available at: http://journals1. scholarsportal.info/details.xqy?uri=/00039993/v88i0009/e70_p2iobtbmhacr.xml. Accessed January 28, 2011.

59. Yang LJ, Gala VC, McGillicuddy JE. Superficial peroneal nerve syndrome: an unusual nerve entrapment. J Neurosurg 2006;104:820–3.

60. Zongzhao L, Jiansheng Z, Li Z. Anterior tarsal tunnel syndrome. J Bone Joint Surg Br 1991;73:470–3.

61. Kuritz HM. Anterior entrapment syndromes. J Foot Surg 1976;15:143–8.

62. Borges LF, Hallett HM, Selkoe DJ, et al. The anterior tarsal tunnel syndrome: report of two cases. J Neurosurg 1981;54:89–92.

63. Garfin S, Mubarak SJ, Owen CA. Exertional anterolateral-compartment syndrome. J Bone Joint Surg 1977;59:404–5.

64. Gessini L, Jandolo B, Pietrangeli A. The anterior tarsal syndrome. J Bone Joint Surg 1984;66A:786–7.
65. Rosselle N, Stevens A. Unexpected incidence of neurogenic atrophy of the extensor digitorum brevis muscle in young normal adults. In: Desmedt JE, editor, New developments in electromyography and clinical neurophysiology, vol. 1. Basel (Switzerland): Karger; 1973. p. 69–70.
66. Dellon AL. Deep peroneal nerve entrapment on the dorsum of the foot. Foot Ankle Int 1990;11:73–80.
67. Allan Maples R, Thom AT, et al. Entrapment of Deep Peroneal Nerve in Dorsal Midfoot Pain. Mississippi Orthopaedic Society Annual Meeting. Greenwood (MS), April 8–10, 2005.

# Tarsal Tunnel Syndrome

John S. Gould, MD[a,b,]*

KEYWORDS

- Tarsal tunnel syndrome • Chronic heel pain
- Space-occupying lesions • Distal tarsal tunnel

Tarsal tunnel syndrome, unlike its similar sounding counterpart in the hand, is a significantly misunderstood clinical entity in every respect. Confusion concerning the anatomy involved, the presenting symptomatology, the appropriateness and significance of various diagnostic tests, conservative and surgical management, and, finally, the variability of reported results of surgical intervention attests to the confusion surrounding this condition. The terminology involved in various diagnoses for chronic heel pain is also a hodgepodge of poorly understood entities, many of which are probably variants of the tarsal tunnel syndrome. Because the diagnosis of carpal tunnel syndrome and its usual causes are well understood, and the name sounds similar to tarsal tunnel syndrome, the diagnostic tools used and the expectations for successful management have not been realized. In fact, the entities have little in common. In the carpal tunnel, the median nerve lies within a fibro-osseous tunnel surrounded by nine tendons, all of which are subject to various inflammatory conditions; also, the underlying carpal bones are subject to synovitis and traumatic dislocations, which create space-occupying lesions. These and hormonal factors result in increased pressure in the tunnel and effects on the nerve, which are easily measurable with delays in nerve conduction and electromyographic changes found in the thenar eminence. These entities do not exist per se in the tarsal tunnel.

## CLASSIC TARSAL TUNNEL SYNDROME

Classic or proximal tarsal tunnel syndrome is the entity to which many clinicians refer, when the term, *tarsal tunnel*, is used. It is an entrapment syndrome of the entire tibial nerve behind the medial malleolus and under the flexor retinaculum or laciniate ligament. The deep and superficial aponeuroses of the leg form the ligament, which is closely attached also to the sheaths of the three adjacent flexor tendons—the

a Section of Foot and Ankle, Division of Orthopaedic Surgery, University of Alabama at Birmingham, 1313 13th Street, South #226, Birmingham, AL 35205, USA
b Division of Orthopaedic Surgery, University of South Alabama, Mobile, AL, USA
* Section of Foot and Ankle, Division of Orthopaedic Surgery, University of Alabama at Birmingham, 1313 13th Street, South #226, Birmingham, AL 35205.
*E-mail address:* Gouldjs@aol.com

Foot Ankle Clin N Am 16 (2011) 275–286
doi:10.1016/j.fcl.2011.01.008
1083-7515/11/$ – see front matter © 2011 Published by Elsevier Inc.

foot.theclinics.com

posterior tibial, the flexor digitorum, and the flexor hallucis. The syndrome was described by Kopell and Thompson[1] in 1960 and then named by both Keck[2] and Lam[3] in 1962.

The clinical presentation is typically of posteromedial pain, tenderness posteromedially over the nerve, a positive Tinel sign in some instances, and in some cases bulging of the retinaculum. In some patients, there may be bona fide neurogenic signs, including both the sensation of numbness and actual hypoesthesia and clawing of the toes. Radiographs, in particular a CT scan, may reveal a lesion, but MRI and/or ultrasound imaging may be more helpful. A nerve conduction study may demonstrate slowing of conduction of the nerve, and electromyography of the intrinsic muscles—abductor hallucis, abductor digiti quinti, and interossei—may also be positive.

Space-occupying lesions have been commonly cited in the cause of this problem. These include ganglia from the subtalar joint or tendon sheaths, lipomas, accessory muscles, tenosynovitis of the adjacent flexors (even though they are within independent sheaths), varicose veins, a bone spicule from an adjacent fracture, foreign bodies. Iatrogenic causes, including osteotomies of the os calcis with inadvertent deep penetration medially or with fixation hardware may be implicated as "lesions." Classic presentations include the following cases.

*A middle-aged physician presented with posteromedial ankle pain, no tenderness, and no neurologic deficits. Radiographs and an initial MRI were obtained. Both were interpreted as negative for pathology. The diagnosis was uncertain and there was little evidence. For more than 2 years, the patient treated himself with analgesics and anti-inflammatory drugs, assuming this to be some form of tendon problem. Although mention was made of tarsal tunnel syndrome, the physical findings were too vague to suggest surgical intervention. Two years later, with symptoms interfering with his work and some complaints of rest pain, another MRI, with greater sensitivity, was done. Again, this was interpreted as normal. With increased interest in ultrasound imaging for assessing nerves, a study with this methodology was done and was interpreted as showing a lipoma lying under the nerve (Fig. 1A). Surgical decompression and excision of the lipoma confirmed the diagnosis and the patient obtained full relief (see Fig. 1B–E). Further review of the MRI reveled that the now obvious lesion had been interpreted as normal fat.*

*A woman in her early 20s presented with a similar history. She was found on MRI and ultrasound imaging to have an accessory muscle, the flexor digitorum accessorious, and had a decompression and excision of the muscle; she had slow but complete relief. We have also removed a small number of ganglions from the tunnel, but these have presented typically more distally and are described later.*

Surgical management of the classic tarsal tunnel and its various causes requires a release of the laciniate ligament and appropriate management of the underlying lesion. Throughout the literature, there are reports of variable outcomes of the surgical procedure, unlike the results of carpal tunnel release, which, although reliable in classic postmenopausal women with the entity, gives variable results in tarsal tunnel release. My opinion and experience with the classic tarsal tunnel outcomes is that when the space-occupying lesion is discrete, as in the cases described previously, and anatomic damage to the nerve does not appear grossly, the anticipation should be for full relief and recovery. When there is obvious damage to the nerve from a fracture or osteotomy, the nerve recovers in a variable manner. When the diagnosis is made without good objective data and the source of compression is not clear, the outcomes are not favorable.

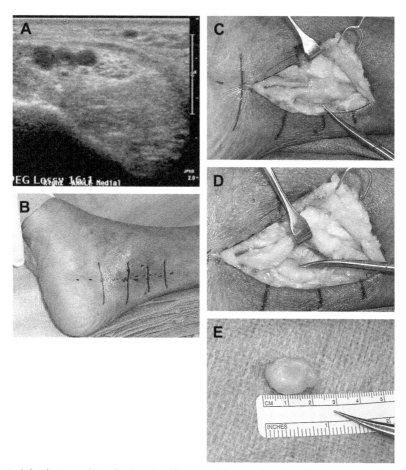

**Fig. 1.** (*A*) Ultrasound study showing lipomas lying under the tibial nerve in the tarsal tunnel. (*B*) Incision marking over classic tarsal tunnel. (*C*) Lipoma (at tip of scissors) lying under the tibial nerve. (*D*) Lipoma dissected from under the nerve. (*E*) Lipoma specimen.

## DISTAL TARSAL TUNNEL SYNDROME

Distal tarsal tunnel syndrome was first described by Heimkes and colleagues[4] in 1987 and is a fairly common entity, especially combined with chronic plantar fasciitis[5] and on occasion with posterior tibial tendon dysfunction.[6] This condition involves irritation to the terminal branches of the tibial nerve, typically the medial plantar, lateral plantar, and medial calcaneal nerves. It may involve combinations of these or only the first branch of the lateral plantar, the nerve to the abductor digiti quinti. The most commonly involved of the branches is the lateral plantar.

### Anatomy

As the tibial nerve travels distally with the posterior tibial artery and vena comitans, it lies plantar to these structures and slightly deeper. The vessels are easily seen just under the laciniate with a darker blue appearance of the veins and a paler blue appearance of the thicker walled artery, lying between the veins. The nerve has a whitish appearance with striations. At variable locations, but typically just under the upper edge of the abductor hallucis muscle, the nerve gives off its various branches (**Fig. 2**).

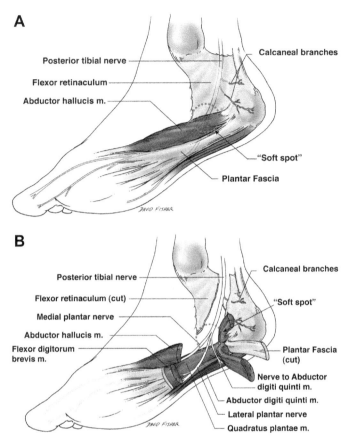

**Fig. 2.** (*A*) Artist's depiction of the tibial nerve passing under the abductor hallucis. (*B*) Artist's depiction of the tibial nerve and branches in the distal tarsal tunnel. Note the soft spot. (*Courtesy of* John S. Gould, MD.)

### Calcaneal branch

Just before passing under the upper edge of the abductor hallucis, the nerve gives off the calcaneal branch or branches, which pass posteriorly, then distally, in the subcutaneous tissue to the skin of the heel. On occasion, the calcaneal branch may emerge under the upper edge of the muscle and then pierce the muscle and its fascia to enter the subcutaneous tissue.

### First branch of the lateral plantar

Just under the upper edge of the abductor, the first branch of the lateral plantar is given off posteriorly. On occasion, it may branch from the lateral plantar portion of the main tibial nerve before the upper edge of the abductor but still travels under the muscle with the lateral plantar. The first branch travels under the abductor hallucis and its deep fascia and over the medial fascia of the quadratus plantae. It passes over the edge of the quadratus fascia and under the medial edge of the plantar fascia, then continues transversely across the heel under the flexor digitorum brevis muscle and sends a sensory branch to the central heel skin, and terminates in the muscle of the abductor digiti quinti.

### Lateral plantar nerve

The lateral plantar nerve continues distally in the tunnel but is more anterior than its first branch, passing under the deep fascia of the abductor hallucis, under the medial edge of the plantar fascia, and over the quadratus plantae and its overlying fascia and then turning distally under the flexor digitorum brevis muscle, emerging under the plantar fascia to form the intermetatarsal nerve to the 4-5 interspace and a branch to the 3-4 intermetatarsal nerve. It also gives off motor branches the intrinsics.

### Medial plantar nerve

The medial plantar nerve emerges typically from the tibial under the abductor hallucis muscle and travels under it with the medial plantar artery and veins, innervating the abductor and then terminating under the plantar fascia into the intermetatarsal nerves to the 1-2, 2-3, and 3-4 interspaces and motor branches to the interossei and lumbricals. In the longitudinal arch subcutaneous tissue, the nerve lies medial to but adjacent to the flexor digitorum and flexor hallucis tendons.

### Pathophysiology

Several causes and mechanisms may create compression of the distal tibial nerve and its branches. A space-occupying lesion, such as a ganglion, may involve the lateral and medial plantar nerves with the lesion emerging from the subtalar or talonavicular joints. A fracture of the medial wall of the calcaneus may cause compression. Neurilemmomas and neurofibromas have been noted to affect these nerves. Direct trauma to the heel and surgical misadventures may affect the calcaneal branches. Inflammatory conditions leading to tenosynovitis of the flexor hallucis and/or flexor digitorum may affect the medial plantar nerve as well as harvesting of the flexor hallucis in this area of the longitudinal arch for a tendon transfer. The more typical cause, however, is traction neuritis of the lateral plantar and first branch of the lateral plantar nerve.

Baxter and Thigpen[7] in 1984 attributed "central heel pad syndrome" in runners to involvement of this nerve branch and suggested release of the deep fascia of the abductor hallucis and medial edge of the plantar fascia to relieve this problem. In this country, this nerve branch is commonly known as Baxter nerve. Rondhuis and Huson[8] in 1986 described what they considered compression of the first branch of the lateral plantar nerve and its association with heel pain. Lau and Daniels,[9] in a cadaver study, demonstrated that with selective division of the supporting structures of the longitudinal arch—the plantar fascia, posterior tibial tendon, and interosseous ligaments—increased traction would occur to the nerve and they suggested traction neuritis as a possible cause of distal tarsal tunnel symptoms in conditions that resulted in arch lowering or collapse. Labib and colleagues[6] in 2002 reported the association with posterior tibial tendon dysfunction. DiGiovanni and Gould, in several reports and publications,[5,10] described the association of distal tarsal tunnel with chronic plantar fasciitis, their approach for decompression, and the outcome of the procedures. The concept for the release is based on this literature suggesting the traction origin.

### History and Physical Findings

The typical patient complaint is pain in the plantar heel, often in the posteromedial aspect of the heel and ankle and sometimes in the longitudinal arch. The history seems similar to plantar fasciitis and is often wrongly diagnosed and treated.

Plantar fasciitis is a distinct entity involving the origin of the plantar fascia on the calcaneus, is an enthesopathy, and presents as such. Pain is experienced in the plantar heel with the first step in the morning or when arising during the day from a resting position. The pain remits after a few steps and does not recur with continued walking. The physical finding is discrete tenderness on the medial tubercle of the calcaneus and essentially there alone. The natural course of that disease is that it is self-limited and that it resolves particularly with stretching exercises, with or without simple over-the-counter arch support.

Tarsal tunnel syndrome, as indicated previously, has a broader area of pain involvement and usually begins with prolonged walking, becoming worse the longer one walks. Unlike plantar fasciitis, the pain does not remit spontaneously or immediately with rest. The pain remits more gradually after non–weight bearing. This more gradual resolution of the pain is described by my colleagues and me as "afterburn." The symptoms may also be even more typically neurogenic, with paresthesias and rest or night pain. These more typical neurogenic symptoms, however, are not always present, although the afterburn typically is. More severe neurologic deficits, such as numbness and/or motor deficits, as manifested by clawing of the toes, are not common with tarsal tunnel syndrome and should bring to mind other diagnoses, including generalized neuropathy, radiculopathy, or central lesions, such as multiple sclerosis.

The physical findings in tarsal tunnel syndrome include point tenderness on the posteromedial heel in the soft spot (**Fig. 3**) at the lower edge of the abductor hallucis where the neurovascular structures enter the foot. As the medial border of the heel is palpated from posteriorly and proximal to distal, the probing finger falls into the soft area (described previously). There may be a Tinel sign over this area and pain may radiate proximally and distally. Palpation of the nerve proximally and in the longitudinal arch may also produce tenderness. In addition, there may be tenderness in each of the intermetatarsal spaces distally, suggesting intermetatarsal neuritis or a Morton neuroma. When the history is of heel pain, however, this distal tenderness represents nerve irritability, not an accompanying distal lesion. If the complaint is of metatarsal pain and the tenderness is also distal, then the lesion is distal as well. With intermetatarsal neuritis or Morton neuroma, the complaint and tenderness are distal but the nerve may also be sensitive proximally or over the soft spot, but the lesion is distal and the patient does not complain of heel pain. This emphasizes the mandatory correlation of the history and the physical.

Distal tarsal tunnel with chronic plantar fasciitis[11] is a common entity and often extraordinarily confusing to clinicians. In truth, it is simpler than it seems. The history and the physical findings combine both entities. The typical history is of plantar fasciitis, which has remitted either with standard noninterventional care or, more typically,

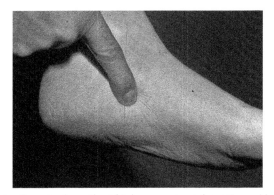

**Fig. 3.** The clinical soft spot where the tibial nerve passes from the ankle to the foot.

with steroid injections to the origin of the plantar fascia. The earlier treatment had been successful, but there is a recurrence. The recurrence may not respond to stretching, injections, or simple inserts.

When the history is carefully obtained, it has changed since the earlier episode. Although there may still be pain with first step in the morning, it may not remit with continued walking or immediately with rest. The afterburn (described previously) may exist. Another presentation is pain with the first step, remission with walking, and then recurrence with prolonged walking and very slow remission of pain afterwards. Finally, there may be rest or night pain, accentuated by pain with first step or walking in general. The physical findings include tenderness over the nerve, over the soft spot, and at the origin of the plantar fascia on the medial tubercle.

Another finding, which validates the impression that this is a traction phenomenon, is that the plantar fascia is attenuated or ruptured. When the ankle is dorsiflexed to neutral or beyond and the great toe is also dorsiflexed, the plantar fascia is placed on stretch. The medial border of the fascia can be palpated with the opposite hand from the metatarsophalangeal joint of the great toe to the heel. When the fascia is attenuated, it becomes less distinct, particularly compared with the normal side, and, in the event of frank rupture, it cannot be felt at all or minimally at best.

### Additional Diagnostic Studies

Imaging studies should be obtained to rule out fractures, in particular stress fractures, or other bone lesions. CT can demonstrate such pathology in more detail. Radioactive isotope bone scanning is nonspecific, leading to a variety of diagnoses, such as stress fractures or osteomyelits, which need correlation with the history and physical and more specific objective testing. MRI is extremely sensitive and shows a space-occupying lesion or a subtle stress fracture that needs to be confirmed with CT. It may also show a defect or thickening in the plantar fascia, suggesting a new or chronic rupture, or simply signal changes at the origin of the plantar fascia, often wrongly interpreted as osteomyelitis or stress fracture, but which may only represent the inflammatory reaction of an enthesopathy. There has been a suggestion that signal changes may be found in nerves with traction neuritis as well, but this has not been a consistent finding (Lopez-Ben R, Department of Radiology, Division of Orthopaedic Surgery, University of Alabama at Birmingham, personal communication, 2010).

Electrodiagnostic studies do not confirm conduction delays nearly as frequently in tarsal tunnel syndrome as with the carpal tunnel syndrome, and a positive test is not considered mandatory for surgical intervention as it is for the upper-extremity condition. Electromyography, however, often shows changes in the abductor hallucis muscle and, when tested, in the abductor digiti quinti.[12] Moreover, the testing is essential when there is any suggestion of generalized neuropathy or radiculopathy. With a strong history and physical findings that correlate with distal tarsal tunnel and the failure of a patient to respond to conservative therapy, a negative electrodiagnostic testing does not provide a contraindication for surgery.

### Nonoperative Treatment

The term, *nonoperative treatment*, rather than *conservative treatment*, is used to suggest that there are indications where surgery rather than a nonoperative approach may be indicated and be the more conservative therapy.

For nonoperative treatment, my colleagues and I use a custom total contact insert with a posteromedial nerve relief channel (**Fig. 4**).[13] The channel is placed in the medial wall of the heel component and to the midline in the plantar area. The channel corresponds to the anatomy of the lateral plantar nerve and its first branch and is placed

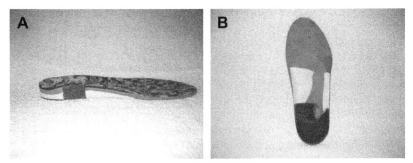

**Fig. 4.** (*A*) Total contact insert with the posteromedial nerve relief channel (medial view). (*B*) Total contact insert with nerve relief channel extending around plantar medial side.

within the cork, which is used for posting the heel and longitudinal arch. The channel is filled with a viscoelastic polymer. When a patient's diagnosis is central heel pad syndrome or the tenderness is also in the central heel pad in distal tarsal tunnel, the channel is extended more posteriorly both medially and plantarward. When the medial plantar nerve seems to be involved, the distal edge of the channel is feathered and the channel may be continued along the medial longitudinal arch. When a distal tarsal tunnel is treated with a more standard insert, without the channel, the patient often states that the insert makes his problem worse. Adding the channel may be dramatic in providing relief. Although there are no hard data to confirm this impression, my colleagues and I think that approximately two-thirds of never-operated patients respond positively to the use of this insert alone. If patients also have residual plantar fasciitis symptoms, my colleagues and I recommend stretching exercises, as described by DiGiovanni and colleagues.[14]

My colleagues and I have used systemic nonsteroidal anti-inflammatory drugs for patients with the plantar fascia component; oral gabapentin and other drugs to ameliorate neurogenic symptoms, with some success; topical anti-inflammatory drugs and nerve pain relievers; and iontophoresis as administered by physical therapy. Patients are urged to avoid modalities, such as heat, cold, and vibration, which are irritating to nerves, negating the use of hot packs, whirlpool baths, and ultrasound, including phonophoresis.

### Operative Intervention

Operative intervention is based on two concepts: (1) treating the residuals of chronic plantar fasciitis and (2) the effort to decompress the tibial nerve and its branches, with emphasis on the lateral plantar and its first branch and the medial calcaneal and the medial plantar when indicated. Medial calcaneal decompression is usually done in recurrent surgery and is discussed in that article by John S. Gould on The Failed Tarsal Tunnel Release. Medial plantar decompression is not routinely done but is discussed. Treatment of the chronic plantar fasciitis component is based on the observation that chronic ruptures of this tissue tend to remain painful with chronic tenderness of the fascia at its origin or with the development of neurogenic symptoms. Complete release of this fascia, as with partial ruptures of other collagen structures, such as tendons (eg, long head of the biceps or flexor carpi radialis), provides relief. The decompression of the nerve is based on the concept of traction of the nerve with the fulcrum of pressure as it passes under the distal edge of the deep fascia of the abductor hallucis and medial edge of the plantar fascia and over the fibers of the quadratus plantae fascia. The nerve can be observed as tented under and over these structures at the soft spot as it makes a significant turn from the ankle into the foot. The releases of the structures allow the nerve to lie freely at this angle.

Because partial rupture of the plantar fascia seems to remain symptomatic, if it is necessary to release some of the plantar fascia to relieve the nerve, my colleagues and I have been hesitant to not release it all. Concern over dorsal arch and lateral border pain after release of the entire plantar fascia has led to a postoperative regimen of non–weight bearing for 4 weeks and the use of the insert postoperatively during the first year. My colleagues' and my experience has shown that this nonweight bearing and use of the insert will obviate the dorsal and lateral foot pain after this procedure.

## Operative Indications

Most patients with a diagnosis of distal tarsal tunnel syndrome with or without chronic plantar fasciitis deserve a trial of nonoperative treatment. If the history and physical are compatible with the diagnosis and there is no indication of radiculopathy or generalized neuropathy or that and other possible diagnoses have been appropriately ruled out, a 6-week trial of treatment with the total contact insert, as described previously, is indicated.

If, at 6 weeks, patients are somewhat improved, this approach is continued for another 6 weeks. As long as improvement is seen, my colleagues and I continue nonoperatively.

If patients are not improved at 6 weeks, initially, the orthotic device is examined to be certain it has been properly made and fits well. Patients are carefully asked if they are using it constantly when up and about. If patients have been compliant and the device is appropriate, diagnostic points are reviewed, and, if still consistent with the initial impression, the surgery is recommended.

If patients were improving with the insert and have reached a plateau, my colleagues and I go through the same procedure and also ask if the patients are satisfied with continuing to use the insert rather than having surgery.

Some patients present with a history and physical totally compatible with the distal tarsal tunnel diagnosis and a significant period of nonoperative treatment, which may be similar to that of my colleagues' and mine but perhaps without the exact regimen. In these cases, I discuss both approaches with the patients. I insist they obtain the type of insert my colleagues and I recommend or modify the one they have to include the nerve relief channel. Patients are usually scheduled for surgery and the insert obtained for them to start to wear. I tell the patients my colleagues and I will proceed as scheduled unless they are so improved with the new inserts that they wish to dolny the surgery

## Operative Technique

The surgery is performed under general or regional anesthesia, but not local, which obscures the anatomy. It is usually an outpatient procedure.[16] A thigh or high calf tourniquet is used along with good lighting and magnifying loupes (3.5× or 4.5×). With the patient in the supine position and the leg externally rotated, a curvilinear incision is begun midway between the posterior edge of the medial malleolus and the medial border of the Achilles tendon. The incision continues distally, curving gently forward to cross the soft spot and then continues across the plantar skin just distal to the heel pad approximately three-fourths of the distance across the plantar surface (**Fig. 5**A).

The vascular bundle is noted under the laciniate ligament. The ligament is divided over the bundle distally to the abductor hallucis superficial fascia, which is also

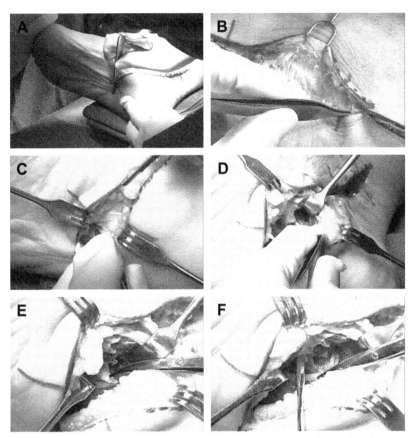

**Fig. 5.** (*A*) The posteromedial incision used for the tarsal tunnel release. (*B*) The laciniate ligament. (*C*) The convex plantar fascia. (*D*) Release of the deep fascia of the abductor hallucis. (*E*) The interval between the abductor hallucis and the flexor digitorum brevis. (*F*) The lateral plantar nerve.

divided, watching for the occasional calcaneal branch, which may pierce it in its proximal substance (see **Fig. 5**B). The subcutaneous fat over the plantar fascia is divided and deeper retractors, such as Senn, are inserted. The convex shape of the plantar fascia is noted and a small angled retractor is placed at the medial edge of the abductor digiti quinti. The entire plantar fascia is divided from the abductor hallucis to the abductor digiti quinti (see **Fig. 5**C).

Dissecting under the abductor hallucis, the muscle is teased away from its deep fascia, approaching the muscle either proximally or distally. A small right angle is inserted into the space between the muscle and fascia, and the deep fascia is divided with tenotomy scissors (see **Fig. 5**D). The division is begun either proximally or distally and then completed from the other direction.

Across from the plantar edge of the abductor hallucis, the muscle of the flexor digitorum brevis is lifted and a deep fascia of variable thickness is also divided. Care is taken throughout this process to avoid lacerating any of the small branches of the posterior tibial artery or veins. If this occurs, I divide the entire abductor hallucis muscle or even the medial edge of the flexor brevis with a cutting cautery to gain good access to the bleeder. To stop this bleeding, I use either bipolar cautery or a small Ligaclip.

Assuming that the incision is properly placed and the abductor is intact, I open the interval between the abductor hallucis and the flexor digitorum brevis with a small self-retaining retractor (Weitlaner) (see **Fig. 5E**). Within this interval are the vascular structures, the first branch of the lateral plantar nerve and the lateral plantar nerve. The first branch lies closer to the posterior heel, the veins with the artery in the middle lie more anteriorly, followed by the lateral plantar nerve, which lies more anteriorly and a little deeper than the vascular structures. Filmy fascia may be found over the nerve, which, with dissection, becomes distinct as a white serrated tubular structure (see **Fig. 5F**).

At this point, the medial plantar nerve has divided off more proximally and is traveling anteriorly under the abductor muscle. Moving the lateral plantar nerve aside with the tip of the tenotomy scissors and a fine forceps, the underlying fibers of the quadratus plantae are visualized and divided.

If the entire abductor hallucis muscle is divided, all of the anatomy is easily visible, but this is not necessary unless vascular access for bleeding is needed; the surgeon is doing a recurrent case that requires full visualization of the nerve; decompression of the medial plantar nerve is required; or the surgeon is disoriented and better visualization of the neurovascular anatomy is needed. I usually do not release the muscle and believe this adds to the morbidity of potentially more scarring.

Additional decompression is done when there is a septum between the vessels and the lateral plantar nerve. This may be seen looking under the abductor muscle and is suspected when seen distally in the interval between the abductor and flexor. The muscle may have to be divided when this is present.

When the medial plantar nerve is involved, I use the same initial approach, divide the muscle, and then, noting exactly where the medial neurovascular bundle is running, make a skin incision over this pathway and decompress the vessels and nerve along this route through the muscle.

The closure consists of dissolving suture (4-0 Monocryl) for the subcutaneous skin of the ankle, with 4-0 nylon on the skin, and skin-only closure with 3-0 nylon for the glabrous skin area plantarly and distally medially.

Postoperatively, the patient is placed in a soft bulky dressing and kept non–weight bearing for the first 2 weeks. Sutures are removed at this time and non–weight bearing is continued for 2 more weeks. No dressing is needed and the patient can bathe the foot. Motion of the foot and toes is encouraged to maintain the gliding of the nerve. At 4 weeks, the patient is allowed to walk with the total contact insert in a shoe or sandal, which is continued for 9 months.

## Outcomes

DiGiovanni and Gould[15] reported an 82% rate of total recovery in a group of primary releases done and followed for at least 2 years, with no recurrences and no patients made worse. In a group of 104 feet in 92 patients operated at the American Sports Medicine Institute, between 1996 and 2000, Hollis and colleagues (Hollis M, Ferguson A, Gould JS, et al. American sports medicine institute review of 104 feet [92 patients] following the complete plantar fascia and tarsal tunnel release between 1996–2000, unpublished data, 2000) found that the average time for patients to reach a plateau of recovery was 19.6 months, with a range of 6 months to 2.5 years. A further report from Gould and DiGiovanni[16] has confirmed continued success with this operative approach with excellent long-term outcomes. The approaches and outcomes related to relapsed, recurrent, or failed procedures are reported by John S. Gould elsewhere in this issue in a subsequent article.

## REFERENCES

1. Kopell HP, Thompson AL. Peripheral entrapment neuropathies of the lower extremity. N Engl J Med 1960;262:56–60.
2. Keck C. The tarsal tunnel syndrome. J Bone Joint Surg Am 1962;44:180–2.
3. Lam SJ. A tarsal tunnel syndrome. Lancet 1962;2:1354–5.
4. Heimkes B, Posel P, Stots S, et al. The proximal and distal tarsal tunnel syndromes: an anatomic study. Int Orthop 1987;11:193–6.
5. DiGiovanni BF, Gould JS. Tarsal tunnel syndrome and related entities. Foot Ankle Clin 1998;3:405–26.
6. Labib SA, Gould JS, Rodriguez del Rio FA, et al. Heel pain triad; the combination of plantar fasciitis, posterior tibial tendon dysfunction, and tarsal tunnel syndrome. Foot Ankle Int 2002;23:212–20.
7. Baxter DE, Thigpen CM. Heel pain: operative results. Foot Ankle 1984;5:16–25.
8. Rondhuis JJ, Huson A. The first branch of the lateral plantar nerve and heel pain. Acta Morphol Neerl Scand 1986;24:260.
9. Lau TC, Daniels TR. Effects of tarsal tunnel release and stabilization procedures on tibial nerve tension in a surgically created pes planus foot. Foot Ankle Int 1998; 19:770–6.
10. DiGiovanni BF, Rodriguez del Rio FA, Gould JS. Chronic disabling heel pain with associated nerve pain: primary and revision surgery results. Podium presentation and abstract at the 17th Annual Summer meeting of the American Orthopaedic Foot and Ankle Society. San Diego, July 2001.
11. Gould JS. Chronic plantar fasciitis. Am J Orthop 2003;32:11–3.
12. Schon LC, Glennon TC, Baxter DE. Heel pain syndrome: electrodiagnostic support for nerve entrapment. Foot Ankle 1993;14:129–35.
13. Gould JS, Ford D. Orthoses and insert management of common foot and ankle problems. In: Schon LC, Porter DA, editors. Baxter's the foot and ankle in sport. Philadelphia: Mosby Elsevier; 2008. p. 585–93. Chapter 27.
14. DiGiovanni BF, Nawoczenski DA, Lintal ME, et al. Tissue-specific plantar fascia stretching exercise enhances outcomes in patients with chronic heel pain. A prospective randomized study. J Bone Joint Surg Am 2003;85(7):1270–7.
15. DiGiovanni BF, Abuzzahab FS, Gould JS. Plantar fascia release with proximal and distal tarsal tunnel release: surgical approach to chronic disabling plantar fasciitis with associated nerve pain. Tech Foot Ankle Surg 2003;2:254–61.
16. Gould JS, DiGiovanni BF. Plantar fascia release in combination with proximal and distal tarsal tunnel release. In: Wiesel SW, editor. Operative techniques in orthopaedic surgery, vol. 4. Philadelphia: Wolters Kluwer/Lippincott Williams and Wilkins; 2011. p. 3911–9. Chapter 57.

# The Failed Tarsal Tunnel Release

John S. Gould, MD[a,b,*]

KEYWORDS

• Tarsal tunnel release • Insufficient release • External scarring
• Intrinsic damage

As noted in the previous article on the tarsal tunnel release, the literature on the tarsal tunnel syndrome presents a confusing picture of the entity itself, the anatomy involved, and the etiology of the condition. While the failure rate ranges from numbers as high as 40% to 60%[1] to the author's data, which suggest numbers as low as less than 5%,[2] this is based on a variety of recommended surgical releases and multiple other factors, to be discussed. In my practice and in that of my associates, large numbers of patients are seen with heel pain and failure to respond to both conservative and surgical measures. As a result of this extensive exposure to the problem over 24 years, the author and colleagues have evolved a series of reasons for surgical failures and potential solutions to these problems.[3] Painful nerves respond to treatment in a variable manner and patients with these problems also have a variety of responses, highly dependent on their own reaction to ongoing painful stimuli. The central perception of pain is a complex process, dependent on multiple factors and various psychological issues that make management of these patients difficult. Nonetheless, the author and colleagues have developed an algorithm for management based on what seem to be logical interpretations of why the nerves remain painful after a surgical release.[4]

## WHY THE SURGICAL RELEASE FAILS

The following are the usual reason for failure of the surgical release:

Inadequate release due to a lack of understanding of the anatomy involved
Failure to execute the release properly
Bleeding with subsequent scarring
Damage to the nerve or its branches in the course of the release
Persistent hypersensitivity of the irritated nerve
Intrinsic damage to the nerve initially.

[a] Section of Foot and Ankle, Division of Orthopaedic Surgery, University of Alabama at Birmingham, 1313 13th Street South, #226, Birmingham, AL 35205, USA
[b] Division of Orthopaedic Surgery, University of South Alabama, Mobile, AL, USA
* Section of Foot and Ankle, Division of Orthopaedic Surgery, University of Alabama at Birmingham, 1313 13th Street South, #226, Birmingham, AL 35205.
E-mail address: Gouldjs@aol.com

Foot Ankle Clin N Am 16 (2011) 287–293
doi:10.1016/j.fcl.2011.03.002
1083-7515/11/$ – see front matter © 2011 Elsevier Inc. All rights reserved

### Inadequate Release Due to the Lack of Understanding of the Anatomy

It is essential to appreciate that although there are space-occupying lesions involved in the classic tarsal tunnel, as described in the prior article, in the so-called distal tarsal tunnel, which the author and colleagues feel is the more common entity, adequate release of the confluence of the superficial and deep fascias of the abductor hallucis and the proximal medial edge of the plantar fascia is essential, as well as the underlying fascia in some cases of the quadratus plantae. As noted in the description of the complete release, the author and colleagues also release the laciniate ligament and the entire plantar fascia. In chronic heel pain, the partial rupture of the plantar fascia is likely a pain generator with persistent symptoms in chronic plantar fasciitis. As nerve pain is also a factor in this entity, the distal, plantar edge of the abductor fascia and medial edge of the plantar fascia appear to be the sites where the nerve sustains the traction irritation.

### Failure to Execute the Release Properly

Landmarks are essential. The soft spot on the posteromedial heel is a distinct location where the neurovascular bundle enters the foot. It marks the exact location of the lateral plantar and where the traction point occurs. The skin incision is made in the midline about halfway between the posterior edge of the medial malleolus and the medial edge of the Achilles tendon. It crosses into the foot over the soft spot (**Fig. 1**A, B) and then extends across the sole of the foot about 3 quarters of the width just distal to the heel pad. As one enters the laciniate ligament, the neurovascular bundle is easily visualized. In the interval between the abductor hallucis muscle and the flexor digitorum brevis, after the fascias have been released, the lateral plantar nerve is found in the distal potion of the tunnel, making a 45° turn in to the plantar foot (see **Fig. 1**C). The first branch of the nerve is more proximal and posterior. If the incision does not follow the surface landmarks, the anatomy is confusing, and

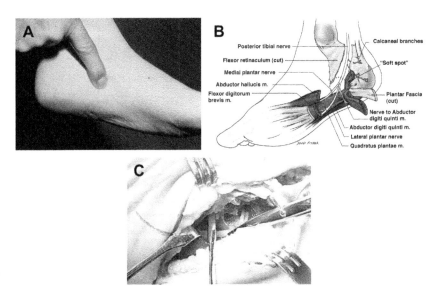

**Fig. 1.** (*A*) The soft spot on the posteromedial heel. (*B*) The anatomy under the soft spot. (*C*) The lateral plantar nerve entering the foot. (*Courtesy of* John S. Gould, MD, with permission.)

the structures are not visualized in this relationship. The release may be inadequate and not include the critical structures.

### Bleeding with Subsequent Scarring

Bleeding not only obscures the visualization of the anatomy, but also leads to increased postoperative scarring and potential traction on the nerve with foot and ankle movement. To avoid this, it is important to use loupe magnification, good lighting, delicate instruments, and careful bipolar cautery. When a vessel is lacerated or torn, and the vena comitans are very vulnerable, I divide the abductor hallucis or flexor digitorum brevis with a unipolar cutting cautery, and use small Ligaclips to halt the bleeding. Careful hemostasis is essential.

### Persistent Hypersensitivity

This problem occurs with neuropathy, and also in some diabetics without neuropathy per se. With longstanding compression/traction and consequent high grades of nerve injury, pain and hypersensitivity may persist. During regeneration of nerves, following release, painful dysesthesia is also not uncommon.

## POTENTIAL SOLUTIONS TO THE CAUSES OF FAILED RELEASES
### Inadequate Releases

Performing an adequate release involves a release of all the structures indicated in the primary release. However, in the revision surgery, I release the abductor hallucis muscle (and possibly the flexor digitorum brevis) with a cutting mode unipolar cautery and fully expose the tibial nerve and its branches, which I do not do in a primary release, where my philosophy is minimal nerve handing, as is recommended with carpal tunnel release. I look for the calcaneal branches, and their possible injury, and for iatrogenic bands crossing the nerve (**Fig. 2**). If there are symptoms involving the medial plantar nerve, the release is carried into the abductor hallucis muscle until the source of compression or irritation is found. Release or external neurolysis alone is done unless damage has occurred to portions of the nerve. If this is found, further measures are taken as described and illustrated.

### External Scarring of the Nerve(s)

The concept of barrier wrapping of nerves in discussed in Dr Masear's article. To summarize, adherence of the nerve to surrounding tissues prevents movement or

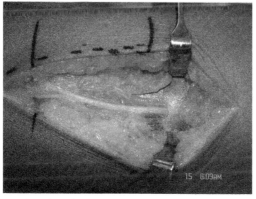

**Fig. 2.** A scar band crossing the tibial nerve.

gliding of the nerve within the tissues as adjacent joints move. As for the tibial nerve, flexion/extension and inversion/eversion of the ankle and subtalar joints require that the nerve moves with these motions. When this gliding fails to occur, due to scarring of the nerve, traction neuritis and pain results. In the natural state, nerves are frequently surrounded by loose adipose tissue. Efforts to replace this gliding tissue have included placing free fat around the nerve and the use of various materials to wrap the nerve. Attempts to wrap rabbit nerves with free fat (Bernard M. O'Brien, MD, Wayne A. Morrison, MD, unpublished data from St Vincent's Microsurgical Unit, Melbourne, Australia, 1982) resulted in the formation of dense adherent fibrous tissue. Free vascularized adipose tissue, muscle ,and fascia have all been used successfully (see Dr Chaudhari's article). Allograft and autograft veins and bovine collagen tubes have all been successfully used in this effort.

The technique for autogenous veins usually involves the use of the greater saphenous vein. The technique involves harvesting the vein, carefully ligating or cauterizing the branches, dissecting free the saphenous nerve, and ligating the ends of the vein on either side of the harvested portion. I usually soak the vein in 1% lidocaine to relax the smooth muscle and then slit it longitudinally. The nerve is wrapped barber pole fashion with the intima of the vein against the nerve. The end of the coil is attached to surrounding tissue and not to the vein itself to avoid a constricting end. The wrapping is done loosely but without redundancy to have enough tissue. The length of graft necessary to wrap a tibial nerve with the greater saphenous is usually about 3 times the length of vein for the length of nerve needing to be wrapped. Each loop is sewn to the adjacent one with 1 or 2 sutures of 6–0 nylon (**Fig. 3**). Gliding seems to occur between the outside of the vein and the surrounding tissues, although there is definitely a tissue plane and some movement between the vein and the nerve (**Fig. 4**).

Collagen tubes are also available for this purpose and are far more convenient. They come in up to 5 cm segments, split longitudinally, and a variety of diameters, ranging from 2 to 12 mm. This allows the nerve to be simply laid within the lumen be rather than to be wrapped. Some brands require a few sutures of 6–0 to close the tube loosely, while other brands open up longitudinally to admit the nerve and wrap around it more than 1 and ½ times so that no sutures are required to close the loop. Segments of various diameters can be applied and then sutured to each other. For example, one might use a larger diameter segment for the tibial nerve and smaller diameters for the lateral and medial plantars. The tube material may also be corrugated to prevent kinking as the nerve goes around a corner (**Figs. 5** and **6**). The advantage of the prepared tubes is the availability in various diameters and quantities, and avoidance of donor site morbidity and scarring. The author's results to date show no difference or advantage of the veins over the commercial products. The bell-shaped curve of outcomes suggests at least 70% significant improvement or relief of pain for all patients in this category with none without some improvement and none made worse.

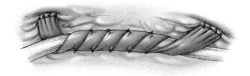

**Fig. 3.** Vein wrapping a nerve. (*Courtesy of* John S. Gould, MD, with permission.)

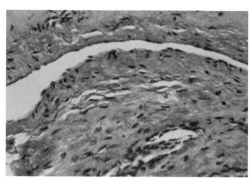

**Fig. 4.** The cleavage plane between the nerve and vein.

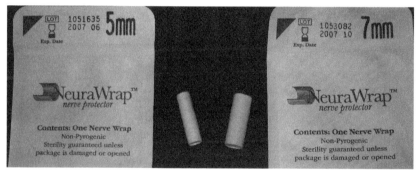

**Fig. 5.** Collagen wraps.

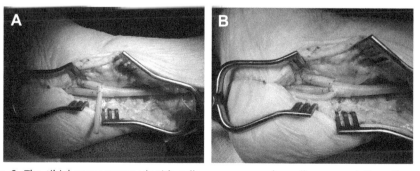

**Fig. 6.** The tibial nerve wrapped with collagen wraps and a collagen conduit on the cut calcaneal nerve. (*A*) The conduit projecting from the nerve. (*B*) The corrugated conduit laid alongside the rest of the wrapped nerve.

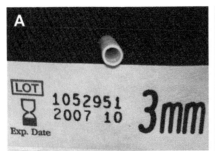
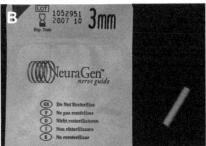

**Fig. 7.** (*A, B*) Collagen conduits.

### Intrinsic Damage to the Nerve

For areas of the nerve with obvious severe internal scar or neuromas in continuity, the author and colleagues had attempted several solutions. When the nerve essentially provides good plantar sensibility, the author and colleagues have wrapped the nerve as described previously, with some success. Neuromas of the calcaneal branches have been placed in vein and collagen conduits (see **Fig. 6**). The author and colleagues have also dissected out, with the microscope, damaged segments; resected them; and grafted with contralateral sural nerve grafts. When the entire tibial or a plantar nerve has been intrinsically damaged and there is no sensibility in its distribution, the author and colleagues have excised the entire segment and repaired with sural graft. When the distal segment is remote or not found, they have placed the end of the nerve within a vein or collagen conduit (see **Fig. 6**; **Fig. 7**). The nerve is drawn into the conduit about 1 cm. A nylon suture is placed on the end of the nerve. A Hewson suture passer is placed through the conduit with the nylon suture ends placed through its loop. The nerve is drawn into the conduit as noted and the edge of the conduit sutured to the epineurium of the nerve with 8–0 monofilament suture using surgical loupes for magnification (**Figs. 8 and 9**).

Collagen conduits are particularly advantageous as they are available in various diameters (eg, 2, 2.5, 3, 4, 5 mm in diameter and 2.5 cm in length). The end of the conduit may be laid next to the parent nerve, or led into a quiet area such as the retro-calcaneal space. The concept of the conduit is that the nerve will regenerate only 1 cm and then fails to form a neuroma with the lack of neurotropic effect of a distal segment of nerve.

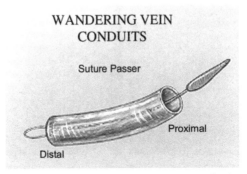

**Fig. 8.** Hewson suture passer within the conduit. (*Courtesy of* John S. Gould, MD, with permission.)

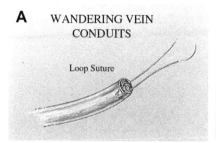
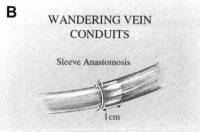

**Fig. 9.** (*A*) The nerve with nylon suture. (*B*) Nerve within the conduit. (*Courtesy of* John S. Gould, MD, with permission.)

Additionally, the author and colleagues have used peripheral nerve stimulators for painful nerves and dorsal column stimulators. At one time, they were fairly enthusiastic about the peripheral nerve stimulators. However, failure to maintain contact of the stimulator electrodes with the nerve, electrical leaks at the stimulator connectors, and other issues including patient complaints of shocking when passing though electronic metal detectors have led to their discontinuation of implantation. Patients are still referred to pain clinic specialists (anesthesiologists) and neurosurgeons who implant dorsal column stimulators. Trial implantations are done routinely before permanent implants. There are many patients with good pain control with these devices, but good studies with reliable data are scanty.

## SUMMARY

Failed surgical releases of the tarsal tunnel may be due to numerous causes including inaccurate diagnosis. Many of the failures are due to lack of appreciation of the involved anatomy or inadequate technique. When an insufficient release is done, a revision simply completes the necessary steps. When external scarring is the problem, barrier materials may be used to help protect the nerve after neurolysis. When intrinsic damage is the problem, either from the primary cause of the lesion or from an iatrogenic etiology, nerve wrapping, reconstruction, conduits, and nerve stimulators all play a role, as indicated, to restore function or ameliorate pain.

## REFERENCES

1. Davies MS, Weiss GA, Saxby TX. Plantar fasciitis: how successful is surgical intervention? Foot Ankle Int 1999;20:803–7.
2. DiGiovanni BF, Abuzzahab FS, Gould JS. Plantar fasciitis release with proximal and distal tarsal tunnel release: surgical approach to chronic disabling plantar fasciitis with associated nerve pain. Tech Foot Ankle Surg 2003;2:254–61.
3. Gould JS. Chronic plantar fasciitis. Am J Orthop 2003;32:11–3.
4. Gould JS, DiGiovanni BF. Plantar fascia release in combination with proximal and distal tarsal tunnel release. In: Wiesel SW, editor. Operative techniques in orthopaedic surgery. Philadelphia: Wolters Kluwer/Lippincott Williams and Wilkins; 2011. p. 3911–9.

# The Painful Neuroma and the Use of Conduits

Emilio Wagner, MD[a,b,c,*], Cristian Ortiz, MD[a,c]

**KEYWORDS**

• Neuroma • Conduit • Graft • Transposition

After nerve injury, a reparative response inevitably takes place, where neurotrophic factors aid axons to regenerate from the proximal stump, and a wallerian degeneration occurs in the distal axon. Degeneration occurs also for a variable distance on the proximal axon. After the period of degeneration, myelinated and unmyelinated fibers grow from the proximal stump, trying to reinnervate the distal stump.[1] If a minimal amount of structures is left of the distal axon, namely, its endoneurial basement membrane, the regenerating fibers reach the end organ. When the complete connective tissue framework is damaged, as in a Sunderland grade IV injury, there is an exaggerated inflammatory response, with extensive deposition of collagen tissue, together with inflammatory cells, and the regenerating fibers do not reach their destination, proliferating in a chaotic manner. The resulting bulb-shaped tissue is known as a neuroma, where an unorganized network of connective tissue is intermingled with nerve fibers, Schwann cells, macrophages, fibroblasts, and myofibroblasts, the latter thought to contribute to pain causing the collagen matrix to contract around nerve fibers.[2] There is a paucity of studies dealing with neuromas in the foot and ankle, and most knowledge comes from level 4 studies, with small numbers of patients involved, and most of them come from hand surgery.

According to the anatomy of peripheral nerves, each nerve is encircled by an external epineurium. Nerve fascicles are group of nerve fibers embedded in endoneurium, correspondingly encircled by perineurium. This structure is the smallest one capable of accepting sutures.[1] Many fascicles are grouped together, surrounded by epineurium, thus forming a classic peripheral nerve. Nerve fibers occupy 25% to

The authors have nothing to disclose.

[a] Universidad del Desarrollo, Escuela de Medicina, Avda Las Condes 12438, Las Condes, Santiago, Chile 7550000

[b] Foot and Ankle Service, Hospital Padre Hurtado, Calle Esperanza 2150, San Ramon, Santiago, Chile 8880465

[c] Foot and Ankle Service, Clinica Alemana, Avda Vitacura 5951, Vitacura, Santiago, Chile 7650568

* Corresponding author. Foot and Ankle Service, Clinica Alemana, Avda Vitacura 5951, Vitacura, Santiago, Chile 7650568.

*E-mail address:* ewagner@alemana.cl

Foot Ankle Clin N Am 16 (2011) 295–304
doi:10.1016/j.fcl.2011.01.004
1083-7515/11/$ – see front matter © 2011 Elsevier Inc. All rights reserved.

foot.theclinics.com

75% of the cross-sectional area of a nerve, compared with the cross-sectional area of a neuroma, which is occupied by 80% of connective tissue.[3] The most common mechanism of nerve injuries are stretch and contusive forces. Common causes include gunshot wounds, fractures, iatrogenic causes, lacerations, and so forth. Classically, nerve lesions have been classified according to Sunderland, where mild lesions with no apparent structural damage are grade I lesions, and grade IV lesions affect all component of the nerve architecture.[1] Every nerve injury, as contusion, avulsion, or direct injury, may produce a neuroma. Neuromas are classified in 3 types: neuromas in continuity, neuromas in completely severed nerves, and amputation neuromas.[2] This article focuses on neuromas in continuity and after completely severed nerves.

## PATHOPHYSIOLOGY

A neuroma alters normal signal conduction through the nerves, and it affects neighboring nerves too. Normal nociceptive responses are augmented, and small stimuli generate abnormal responses, creating, for example, hyperesthesia. This hyperexcitability may be explained by an abnormal accumulation of potassium ion channels and sodium ion channels on the axons in the neuroma.[3] This hyperexcited state explains what has been called ectopic neuralgia, where a patient suffers spontaneous pain discharges without any external stimulus.[4] Locally, the disorganized connective and neural tissue, where the nerve fibers innervate scar tissue and skin, yield neuromas sensitive to mechanical stimulation.[5] This has been called nociceptive neuralgia.[4]

## PATIENT EVALUATION

A complete understanding of the neural anatomy in the foot and ankle is needed to understand and interpret symptoms and clinical signs. A review of the pertinent anatomy is beyond the scope of this article, but it is recommended for understanding how to proceed with neuroma treatment. The mechanism of injury is important, because it is different when dealing with a gunshot wound or an open fracture, where nerve scarring is expected, a gradual decrease in nerve function may be observed, and a longer waiting time before intervention is warranted, compared with a clean, sharp injury where immediately afterwards a deficit in nerve function appears and a sooner operative intervention is recommended.

Pain in relation to a surgical scar which also radiates along the course of a nerve is a typical clinical sign of a neuroma. There may be a Tinel sign on top of the scar and altered sensation in the territory corresponding to that specific nerve. The authors agree with Mackinnon in that patients who are willing to palpate and massage the area of pain are not good surgical candidates. The area of discomfort should be painful to light touch, and pain proximal to the suspected area of neuroma is a frequent finding (sometimes called "Mackinnon sign") and should be looked for.[3] The complete area and its surroundings should be inspected and palpated to find additional territories innervated by nerves which may be involved in the neuropathic pain. These additional nerves have to be addressed when performing a surgical intervention.

Imaging studies generally are not necessary, except when dealing with previous open multiple fractures or gunshot wounds, where the exact location of the injury is not completely clear. Ultrasound imaging may assist in being certain where the lesion is. An MRI can also be obtained, although its utility is best when dealing with bone or soft tissue tumors, if no history of injury is clear. A history of chronic symptoms may indicate the need for an electrodiagnostic study. This study is also useful when following the recovery of an injured nerve. Diabetes and hypothyroidism have to be ruled out, because they are common systemic disorders that may present with neuropathic pain of unknown origin.

## TREATMENT

When dealing with a severed nerve, the ideal treatment is a primary direct repair. If that is not possible, a reconstruction using some sort of nerve conduit or nerve grafting is the procedure of choice. A nerve repair provides an adequate environment for the proximal regenerating axons to find their way into the distal stump and reach their final organ destination. The use of grafts or absorbable or artificial nerve conduits also provide an environment for regenerating axons. For this regeneration process to happen, we have to achieve ideal local conditions for which a clear knowledge of the regional anatomy and magnification loupes are needed. To help decrease local scarring a minimum amount of sutures should be used besides obtaining a tension-free repair.[1]

If there already is a neuroma, either in a severed nerve or a neuroma in continuity, how critical the function is of the nerve that is worked with and what the consequences are if the nerve is deleted need to be known. The authors consider nerve function to be critical if its loss will hinder in some way the normal foot function: losing motor function important for normal daily activities (losing intrinsic muscle function in the foot, which may create hammer or claw toe deformities, or losing extrinsic muscle function, as in a common peroneal nerve injury) or losing protective sensation in the sole of the foot that renders an insensate foot with the known risks of ulcerations. After analyzing how critical the function of the injured nerve is, we can plan the necessary intervention.

Before surgery, a trial of conservative treatment is warranted, even though the benefits of it are inconsistent.[6,7] Available alternatives include cryotherapy, desensitization therapies, therapeutic nerve blocks, transcutaneous electrical nerve stimulation, local use of capsaicin-derived gels, oral medications that decrease neuropathic pain as pregabalin or gabapentin, acupuncture, and so forth. If these treatments fail, a surgical intervention is planned.

Simple resection has been used by many surgeons, but there is evidence in the literature that neuroma resection is not routinely successful.[6] The reported reoperation rates have been as high as 65%, which explains the use of additional maneuvers, such as burying the proximal stump into some other tissue.

Generally speaking, if dealing with critical nerves, such as the tibial or common peroneal nerve, the treatment of a neuroma is nerve or conduit grafting. If the nerve is not critical, then a neuroma resection and transfer to a muscular bed is the method of choice (**Figs. 1 and 2**).[3,5–8]

## APPROACH TO INJURED NERVES WITH CRITICAL FUNCTION

Critical nerves are the main tibial nerve and the common peroneal nerve. If the entire tibial nerve is injured, there is pain at the injury site with lack of sensation and motor function on the distribution of the tibial nerve, posterior tibial muscle, hallux and toe flexors, and intrinsic muscles, as well as loss of sensibility on the plantar aspect of the foot. This lack of sensation is badly tolerated and may result in skin breakdown and ulcerations. This skin breakdown is more likely to occur if there are associated foot deformities. For the peroneal nerve, lack of sensation in the dorsum of the foot and lack of motor function corresponding to the lateral and anterolateral compartments of the leg are seen. A nerve reconstruction should be attempted, extending the previous surgical scar proximally to find a healthy nerve and distally past the neuroma. A resection of the neuroma and a nerve graft should be used. Most

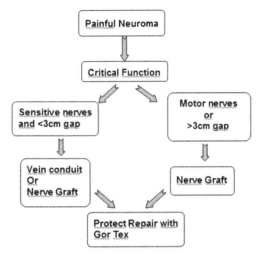

**Fig. 1.** Decision-making diagram for critical nerves.

commonly, the contralateral sural graft is used, taking care to dissect the nerve and its branches to get the maximum donor tissue. The reconstruction has to be tension-free, and epineurial sutures should be used.[3,5,7] A trend toward using bioabsorbable conduits has been observed in the last two years. Good results have been shown for sensory nerves, especially for gaps under 3 cm in length.[9] For motor nerve reconstruction, good results have been shown, but a better prognosis is found for the tibial than for the peroneal nerve.[10]

If no proximal stump is available, a nerve transfer can be performed using the sural nerve or the superficial peroneal nerve. These last two nerves are transected distally, taken to the medial side, performing an end-to-end repair with the medial or lateral plantar branch and an end-to-side repair of the remaining distal branches of the donor into the intact proximal portion of the transferred donor nerve (an epineurotomy window is provided on the donor).[3]

When dealing with the distal branches of the tibial nerve, that is, the calcaneal, medial plantar, or lateral plantar nerves, the authors strive to preserve plantar sensibility and, therefore, perform graft reconstruction for medial or lateral plantar nerve

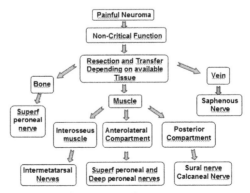

**Fig. 2.** Decision-making diagram for noncritical nerves.

injuries. After reconstruction, the graft is protected and the neighboring nerve ends with a nonabsorbable conduit, expanded polytetrafluoroethylene (Preclude Spinal Membrane [Gore & Associates, Flagstaff, AZ, USA]), which has decreased the rate of postsurgical scarring around the reconstruction (Cristian Ortiz, MD, Emilio Wagner, MD, unpublished data, 2010) (**Fig. 3**). If the calcaneal branch is damaged, it is considered a noncritical function nerve, and thus, it is dissected and transposed proximally into a different tissue bed (discussed later). If the grafting fails for the medial or lateral plantar nerves, the authors recommend resecting the neuroma, dissecting it proximally from the main posterior tibial trunk, and transposing it into the soleus muscle.[3]

## APPROACH TO INJURED NERVES WITHOUT CRITICAL FUNCTION

For these type of nerves, because the resulting deficit in function is mild and the denervation if a nerve is resected is well tolerated, no reconstruction is attempted. A reconstruction will have a longer recovery time and the surgical effort won't be rewarded with an equal return in function. As discussed previously, simple resection of a neuroma does not suffice in the majority of cases, and, therefore, most investigators recommend adding a transfer of the nerve to a tissue bed, which hopefully will decrease mechanical and neurotrophic stimuli to avoid painful neuroma formation, provided that this tissue bed is nonmobile or has little mobility and gives adequate mechanical cushioning. Most articles refer to transposing nerves to muscle beds,[3–7,11–14] with reported success rates of 80%. In animal models, nerve ends in muscle beds form rounded smooth bulbs with well-organized nerve fibers nonadherent to surrounding tissue.[6]

Other options have been studied as tissue beds for injured nerves. Translocating nerves into veins has been reported, with 87% satisfaction, although in a small case series.[15] In this series, the nerve stump was transposed into a vein in an end-to-end fashion, or in an end-to-side fashion, or into a vein which was then tied distally.[6] The article suggests that this option could be better done for smaller sensory nerves. Its advantage is that it uses local freely available tissue, obviating extending the incision in search for muscular or bone tissue as alternatives. Another option using local veins is called the extended autologous venous nerve conduit, referencing the action of transposing a nerve into a vein and the vein burying into a muscle.[6]

Translocating the nerve ends into bone is another alternative studied. Results ranging from 70% to 90% success rates are reported in the literature, all small case

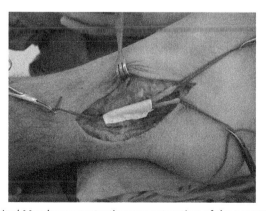

**Fig. 3.** Preclude Spinal Membrane protecting reconstruction of the posterior tibial branches (plantar medial and lateral).

series.[6] Chiodo and Miller[16] showed a 75% satisfaction rate for superficial peroneal neuromas translocated into the fibula compared with a 46% rate for relief of symptoms when transposed into the peroneus brevis muscle.

Finally, nerve-to-nerve anastomosis has been reported, either end-to-end or end-to-side anastomosis. The results reported are good, although in very small series.[6,17]

The authors' surgical alternative depends on the nerve and the surrounding tissue (see **Fig. 1**). Generally speaking, when dealing with the superficial peroneal nerve, the authors try to resect the neuroma and translocate it into bone or lateral compartment musculature. For the deep peroneal nerve, calcaneal branch of the posterior tibial nerve, intermetatarsal nerve, saphenous nerve, and sural nerve, the authors try to bury into the nearest muscle, which provides a good resting bed. If the muscle is considered too far away from the neuroma, or, if after resection the proximal stump of the nerve is considered too short, a venous conduit is used, using the vein to route the nerve into a muscular area.

## APPROACH TO INDIVIDUAL NERVES
### Calcaneal Nerve Neuroma

A neuroma of this nerve can be seen after plantar fasciotomy, calcaneal spur removal, or tarsal tunnel decompression,[12] the latter of these the most common in the authors' practice. The surgical approach should be an extension of the previous surgical incision, generally the tarsal tunnel incision after the posterior tibial nerve. The incision has to be extended proximally and distally if necessary. After identification of the neuroma, it is resected and translocated proximally into the nearest muscle belly, typically the flexor hallucis longus (**Fig. 4**). Although this approach has good reported results, the flexor hallucis longus may not provide adequate protection because it is a very mobile muscle. The authors try, if possible, to additionally protect the nerve with a vein conduit.

### Intermetatarsal Nerve Neuromas

Intermetatarsal nerve neuromas result from an inadequate initial approach to an intermetatarsal neuritis, or Morton neuroma. After initial surgery for a true neuroma of these nerves, the authors favor a plantar longitudinal approach, starting at the level of the metatarsal head distally, which provides good exposure and the possibility of extending the incision proximally if needed (**Fig. 5**). A dorsal approach could be used if clear signs of a totally inadequate previous dissection are present as a short nerve reported in the previous biopsy or an extremely short dorsal incision. After dissecting through

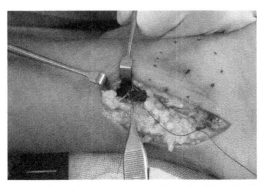

**Fig. 4.** Transposition of a calcaneal nerve neuroma into the flexor hallucis longus muscle.

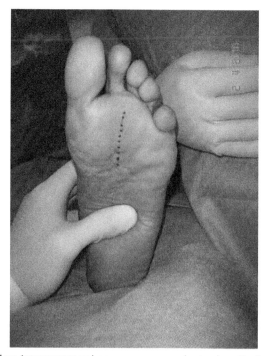

**Fig. 5.** Revision of an intermetatarsal nerve neuroma, plantar longitudinal approach.

the plantar fascia, the corresponding branches of the medial or lateral plantar nerves are identified, the neuroma is resected, and the proximal stump is tagged with absorbable suture and passed through the interosseus muscles to the dorsum of the foot (**Fig. 6**). The suture is attached to the subcutaneous layer of the dorsum of the foot, allowing the nerve to rest approximately 1 cm below the skin level. If left with a small proximal stump after resecting the neuroma, specifically when too near to a proximal division of the main trunk of the nerve (medial plantar or lateral plantar nerve), the authors use a vein conduit to protect the nerve stump, suture it through the epineurium to the vein, and pass a suture through the distal end of the vein and pass it to the dorsum, suturing it to the dorsal subcutaneous layer, taking care to leave the free end of the vein 1 cm below the level of the skin.

Although it has not been the authors' experience, it has been suggested that many of these cases may have a concomitant tarsal tunnel syndrome, which should be ruled out before deciding the specific plan for surgery.[14] This entity may be suspected if multiple sites of neuropathic pain are present with just one surgery done previously or if the pain is present in an atypical intermetatarsal space. In these cases, other causes should be ruled out as systemic causes of neuropathic pain (discussed previously). A neuroma in the second intermetatarsal space may cause tenderness or have some referral of pain to the first intermetatarsal space; the third intermetatarsal space neuroma may cause symptoms in the fourth intermetatarsal space. Because primary neuromas are unusual in these spaces (first or fourth intermetatarsal space), imaging, including MRI and ultrasound, may be indicated to confirm the lack of pathology in these spaces. In addition, patients with tarsal tunnel syndrome complain of pain in the heel and arch but may be sensitive in all the intermetatarsal spaces. Furthermore, patients with intermetatarsal neuromas complain of pain in the metatarsal region both

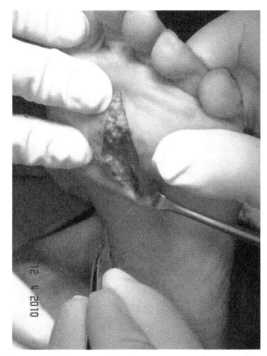

**Fig. 6.** Tagging of the proximal stump of an intermetatarsal nerve after neuroma resection before passing it to the dorsum of the foot.

dorsally and plantarly while also exhibiting sensitivity on testing over the tibial nerve posteromedially at the heel. These observations may lead to confusion if the history is not carefully taken or these facts are not appreciated.

### Sural Nerve Neuroma

Sural nerve neuroma may occur after sural nerve biopsies, which is the most frequent cause seen by the authors. The previous surgical scar should be extended longitudinally following the course of the nerve. An additional incision may be used proximally to recover the nerve on the posterior aspect of the calf, to translocate the nerve into a muscular bed, generally between the gastrocnemius or soleus muscle.[5] The authors' preferred method currently is to transpose the nerve into a local vein in an end-to-end fashion, as suggested by Koch and colleagues,[15] because it allows decreasing the size of the surgical incision.

### Saphenous Nerve Neuromas

Injury to the saphenous nerve may occur after saphenous vein harvest for cardiac surgery or, more frequently in the authors' center, after orthopedic procedures, namely, ankle fracture treatment. The incision should be placed longitudinally following the nerve direction. The neuroma has to be resected and transposed into the leg as proximal as possible. The authors have tried translocating the nerve into the tibia with success but only in few cases (Emilio Wagner, MD, Cristian Ortiz, MD, unpublished data, 2009). If the neuroma is near the ankle, in young women or patients with high cosmetic expectations, the authors do not extend the incision more proximal to transpose it to muscle and use a vein conduit to protect it and hopefully reach

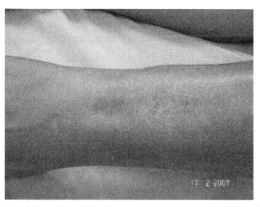

**Fig. 7.** Anterior aspect of the ankle joint showing scar result of previous distal tibia fracture, with superficial peroneal neuroma symptoms.

a muscular bed.[15] If the neuroma is proximal to the ankle, a transfer of the proximal stump to the posterior musculature is possible.

### Superficial Peroneal Nerve

The superficial peroneal nerve may be injured in the lower leg when fasciotomies are performed at the level of the ankle when fractures are addressed or in the anterior part of the ankle when ankle arthroscopies are done (**Fig. 7**). A Tinel sign is present, and pain and numbness in relation to the territory innervated by the corresponding branch are present. When the neuroma is present proximal to the ankle, a resection of the neuroma and a translocation of the nerve to the lateral muscular compartment is the rule.[3] Transposing it into the fibula is another alternative with good reported results.[16] When present at the level of the ankle, an extended longitudinal incision should be done to translocate the proximal stump proximally into the anterior muscular compartment. When using either muscular compartment, a fasciotomy of the corresponding compartment has to be done, because it prevents recurrence of pain decreasing the pressure of the new nerve environment.[13]

### SUMMARY

Treatment of neuromas in the foot and ankle is evolving. There is a paucity of studies dealing with neuromas in this anatomic region and most knowledge comes from hand surgery. A trend toward reconstructive surgery using nerve grafts and conduits for nerves with critical function is being seen, including the use of artificial conduits for motor nerves. For noncritical nerves, the most generally accepted treatment is neuroma resection and burial into a tissue bed, commonly muscle, which protects the proximal stump and avoids the generation of a painful neuroma. A clear knowledge of the neural anatomy is paramount together with correct identification of all the nerves involved in the pain generation process. More studies dealing with neuromas in this area are needed to provide evidence-based information.

### REFERENCES

1. Midha R, Mackay M. Principles of nerve regeneration and surgical repair. Semin Neurosurg 2001;12(1):81–92.
2. Mavrogenis A, Pavlakis K, Satamatoukou A, et al. Current treatment concepts for neuromas-in-continuity. Injury 2008;39:43–8.

3. Vernadakis A, Koch H, Mackinnon S. Management of neuromas. Clin Plast Surg 2003;30:247–68.
4. Vora A, Schon L. Revision peripheral nerve surgery. Foot Ankle Clin 2004;9(2): 305–18.
5. Mackinnon S. Neuromas. Foot Ankle Clin 1998;3(3):385–404.
6. Wu J, Chiu D. Painful neuromas: a review of treatment modalities. Ann Plast Surg 1999;43(6):661–7.
7. Glazebrook M, Paletz J. Treatment of posttraumatic injuries to the nerves in the foot and ankle. Foot Ankle Clin 2006;11:183–90.
8. Lewin-Kowalik J, Marcol W, Kotulska K, et al. Prevention and management of painful neuroma. Neurol Med Chir (Tokyo) 2006;46:62–8.
9. Moore A, Kasukurthi R, Magill C, et al. Limitations of conduits in peripheral nerve repairs. Hand (N Y) 2009;4:180–6.
10. Rosson G, Williams E, Dellon A. Motor nerve regeneration across a conduit. Microsurgery 2009;29:107–14.
11. Nahabedian M, Johnson C. Operative management of neuromatous knee pain: patient selection and outcome. Ann Plast Surg 2001;46:15–22.
12. Kim J, Dellon A. Neuromas of the calcaneal nerves. Foot Ankle Int 2001;22(11): 890–4.
13. Dellon A, Aszmann O. Treatment of superficial and deep peroneal neuromas by resection and translocation of the nerves into the anterolateral compartment. Foot Ankle Int 1998;19:300–3.
14. Wolfort S, Dellon A. Treatment of recurrent neuroma of the interdigital nerve by implantation of the proximal nerve into muscle in the arch of the foot. J Foot Ankle Surg 2001;40(6):404–10.
15. Koch H, Hubmer M, Welkerling H, et al. The treatment of painful neuroma on the lower extremity by resection and nerve stump transplantation into a vein. Foot Ankle Int 2004;25(7):476–81.
16. Chiodo C, Miller S. Surgical treatment of superficial peroneal neuroma. Foot Ankle Int 2004;25(10):689–94.
17. Lidor C, Hall R, Nunley J. Centrocentral anastomosis with autologous nerve graft treatment of foot and ankle neuromas. Foot Ankle Int 1996;17(2):85–8.

# Interdigital Neuralgia

Paul G. Peters, MD, Samuel B. Adams Jr, MD, Lew C. Schon, MD*

**KEYWORDS**

- Interdigital neuroma • Interdigital neuralgia • Morton's neuroma
- Morton's metatarsalgia

Historical descriptions of conditions related to the fourth toe date back to 1835. In Larson and colleagues'[1] description of the historical perspectives of forefoot neuromas, the first written account is ascribed to Civinini, a professor of anatomy at the University of Pisa.[2] He identified a fusiform swelling in the common plantar digital nerve of the third interspace. Durlacher, the Queen's Surgeon-Chiropodist, wrote of an affliction in the forefoot affecting the plantar nerve, and is credited with the first clinical report.[1] Morton later hypothesized that there was a problem related to the fourth metatarsophalangeal (MTP) joint with involvement of the lateral plantar nerve (LPN). In his original paper, he summarized the treatment of 16 patients. Three patients had a resection of the fourth MTP joint and nerves and 1 toe amputation with successful results. The remaining patients were treated with local blood-letting, anodyne applications, and rest until symptoms resolved.[1] In 1893, Hoadley[3] explored the painful area and excised a small neuroma and reported a "prompt and perfect cure." Tubby,[4] in 1912, observed two patients with congested and thickened digital plantar nerves. "Morton's metatarsalgia is a neuritis of the fourth digital nerve" said Betts in 1940.[5] McElvennhy[6] stated it was caused by a tumor in the most lateral branch of the medial plantar nerve. Compression by the deep intermetatarsal ligament has also been hypothesized. Gauthier[7] reported good clinical outcomes with release alone, in 1979, and was then supported with anatomic studies.[8,9] A more detailed historical prospective is presented by Kelikian[10] and Larson and colleagues.[1]

## ANATOMY AND PATHOLOGY

Nomenclature for interdigital neuroma is historically based and misleading. Histologic analysis does not indicate a true nerve tumor.[9,11] Interdigital neuritis, suggested by Weinfeld and Myerson,[12] is also inexact because the suffix "-itis" implies inflammation.

---

No funding was received for this study.

The authors have nothing to disclose.

Department of Orthopaedic Surgery, Foot and Ankle Service, Union Memorial Hospital, 3333 North Calvert Street, Suite 400, Baltimore, MD 21218, USA

* Corresponding author.

*E-mail address:* lewschon@comcast.net

The best terminology would be interdigital neuralgia (IDN), because of the predominance of pain symptoms and the lack of inflammation.

The etiology of this condition remains unclear. Multiple histologic reports described intraneural fibrosis, sclerohyalinosis in the interstitium, increased elastic fibers in the stroma, and degeneration of nerve fibers without signs of Wallerian degeneration.[8,9,11] Lassmann[9] and Graham and Graham[8] localized these changes to always being distal to the transverse metatarsal ligament, supporting the theory of entrapment neuropathy. However, Morscher and colleagues[13] performed nerve biopsies on typical patients with IDN and compared them to asymptomatic nerves biopsied at autopsy. They confirmed histologic epineurial and perineurial fibrosis but were unable to show a significant difference between IDN biopsies and autopsy neuroma excision. Another anatomic study examined the distance of the common digital nerve bifurcation to the deep transverse metatarsal ligament (DTML) during 2 phases of the gait cycle. They then compared the location of excised neuromas to the bifurcation, concluding that neuromas remain distal to the DTML during the normal gait cycle, specifically at midstance and heel-off.[14] Other factors should be considered, including anatomic, mechanical, traumatic, and extrinsic factors.

Anatomically, variations in metatarsal head spacing, the obliquity of the intermetatarsal ligament after a metatarsal shaft fracture, terminal nerve branching, and mobility of the surrounding joints may contribute to this neuralgia. The plantar foot is supplied by the lateral plantar nerve (LPN) and medial plantar nerve (MPN). The MPN branches into the first, second, and third common digital nerves, supplying the concomitant web spaces. LPN branches into a common digital nerve to the fourth interspace and a proper digital nerve to the lateral side of the small toe. A communicating branch between the third and fourth common digital nerves is present in approximately 27% to 28% of feet.[15,16] Levitsky and colleagues[16] additionally observed that the second and third interspace were significantly more narrow in comparison with the first and fourth, possibly contributing to compression.

The mobility differential between the medial 3 rays and the fourth and fifth rays has also been proposed as a contributing factor. The first, second, and third metatarsals are relatively well fixed to the cuneiform complex, whereas the fourth and fifth metatarsals' articulation with the cuboid are much more mobile. In crossing this transition zone, the common digital nerves are potentially exposed to traction and trauma. Alternatively, the increased movement may induce an enlarged bursa, venous congestion, or compression of the nerve resulting in IDN. However, the considerable incidence of second interspace neuromas negate this as the primary cause.[17]

A direct insult to the nerve occasionally results in the origin of an IDN, such as stepping on a sharp object, crush, or an acute traction injury. Repetitive microtrauma from prolonged standing or walking especially on hard surfaces with uncushioned shoes may be causative. This overuse is also plausible in runners, dancers, or athletes who posture, run, spin, cut, or jump with high forefoot forces, which are likely aggravating factors for the condition. In this same population, excessive dorsiflexion of the MTPs can further add to symptoms and signs. Fat pad atrophy to varying degrees will make the nerve more vulnerable to injury. Extrinsic forces, such as an MTP joint ganglion, plantar lipoma, MTP joint instability, or thickened transverse metatarsal ligament can cause interdigital neuralgia. Occasionally, the transverse metatarsal ligament is thickened or contains an aberrant band, which, when released, resolves the neuralgia.[18] MTP joint capsule attenuation allows medial deviation of the third toe, which in turn forces the third metatarsal head laterally, reducing the third interspace volume and clinically results in neuroma symptoms in approximately 10% to 15% of patients.[18] This ligament attenuation may permit traction on the nerve as well. Plantar plate disruption can allow for MTP mal-position, subluxation, or dislocation, all of which can strain the nerve. Thickening of the MTP joint owing to capsulitis, synovitis, or arthritis can irritate the nerve as well. Fracture and its sequelae of malunion or nonunion also can conceivable alter the interspace volume from stress or trauma, with the additional potential of a traumatic neuroma from a crush or twisting mechanism. Finally, patients with diffuse or more proximal nerve pathology are more vulnerable to manifest with nerve symptoms from any of the previously mentioned etiologies.

## HISTORY AND PHYSICAL EXAMINATION

The reported average age of presentation is 55 years (29 to 81 years) with an increased prevalence in women (4 to 15 times).[17,19] The primary complaint is pain localized to the plantar forefoot between the metatarsal heads. The symptom complex is typically described as sharp, stabbing, burning, electric, or tingling with radiation to the toes. Patients often complain of a fullness under the toes or the feeling of "the wadding up of their sock" under the toes. Occasionally, the pain radiates to the dorsum of the foot or more proximally along the plantar aspect of the foot.

Unilateral symptoms predominate with a 15% incidence of bilateral neuromas. Two neuromas occurring simultaneously in one foot was reported to be less than 3%.[20] The most common location is the third web space by most reports. Hauser[21] noted an equal distribution between the second and third web spaces, which was not supported by Graham and colleagues.[22] An IDN in the first or fourth interspace is very unusual and may not exist as a clinical entity.

The typical patient complains that symptoms are exacerbated by tight-fitting high-heeled or dress shoes, with relief upon removal and rubbing the foot. Patients may also avoid rolling through the ball of the foot or voluntarily curl their toes during the gait cycle to limit pain symptoms. The use of a wide-cushioned thick-soled walking or jogging shoe can significantly mitigate symptoms. Recently, the well-marketed, "over-the-counter" stiff rocker-soled shoes have provided some relief. However, if symptoms have been present for longer than 12 months, the benefits of many nonoperative treatment modalities may be significantly negated.

The physical examination is performed to look for evidence of the neuroma and to rule out other pathology. The foot alignment must be assessed while standing, to detect deviation or clawing of the toes or swelling or fullness of the web spaces in comparison with the contralateral foot. The skin is inspected for intractable plantar keratosis, erythema, or calluses. Next, the MTP joints are evaluated, which includes the assessment of range of motion, synovitis, plantar fat pad pain, and joint stability. An MTP drawer test is important, especially in the second toe, not only to assess for tenderness, but to confirm joint stability.

Typically, plantar palpation of the web spaces reproduces the pain associated with interdigital neuralgia. During the examination, it is important to start proximally along the medial and lateral plantar nerves and then proceed distally to the common digital nerves. Carefully delineate the difference between pain along the metatarsal head and its capsular structures versus the interspace that contains the nerve. Of critical importance is to avoid inadvertent extraneous dorsal pressure, which may trigger pain unrelated to tender plantar structures.

Additionally, with application of mediolateral pressure to the metatarsal heads, the presence of a mechanical sensation such as a "clunk," "crunch," or "click" and reproduction of the pain (Mulder's sign) is considered supportive of an IDN.[23] The presence of the mechanical sensation without the pain can be a normal finding.

The tibial nerve and all of its branches are palpated and percussed. The sural, saphenous, deep peroneal, and superficial peroneal nerves should be evaluated as well. A gross motor examination, reflexes, and straight leg raise are also performed. Lumbar spine radiculopathy has the ability to create a similar presentation and occult compression may make the common plantar nerves more sensitive to compression or irritation (double crush phenomenon). Repeat clinical examination during the same visit or on a subsequent evaluation can be extremely helpful to confirm that an IDN is indeed the diagnosis.

The patient's shoe wear, both occupational and social, is evaluated, because 90% of women wear shoes that are too tight. Many fashionable shoes have a minimal sole and stay on by forefoot compression alone. As suggested by Kay and Bennett,[24] trace the patient's foot while standing and then place the shoe over the tracing to demonstrate the number of toes not contained in the toe box. In addition, a high heel will drive pressures to the forefoot and the relative dorsiflexion of the MTPs will stretch the IDN further.

The reported physical findings from Mann's clinical practice include plantar tenderness, 95%; radiation of pain into the toes, 46%; palpable mass, 12%; numbness, 3%; and widening of the interspace, 3%.[18]

### Diagnostic Studies

Anteroposterior (AP), lateral, and oblique weight-bearing foot radiographs are obtained to evaluate for subluxation, dislocation, arthritis, or any other osseous abnormality. The use of MRI and ultrasound for diagnosis is controversial. Sharp and colleagues[25] concluded that reliance on either MRI or ultrasound would have led to an inaccurate diagnosis in 18 of 19 cases. Clinical evaluation alone provided a more accurate assessment. Ultrasound does have its proponents with reports of up to 92% accuracy,[26] but is operator dependent.[27] Bencardino and colleagues[28] reported an asymptomatic incidence of "IDN" to be 33%, based on a blinded retrospective review of 57 MRIs of the foot. We do not feel MRI or ultrasound is useful in the diagnosis of IDN. If one is suspicious of other etiologies, such as a stress fracture or soft tissue mass, they may be of some benefit.

Standard electrodiagnostic studies are not beneficial in the diagnosis of interdigital neuralgia. Almeida and colleagues[29] demonstrated an abnormal dip phenomenon as a characteristic for diagnosis using near-nerve needle nerve conduction. Generally, electrodiagnostic studies are not indicated unless one suspects radiculopathy or more proximal nerve compression.

Diagnostic injections with local anesthetic can be beneficial, but may be nonspecific with pain relief to other local pathology. Despite local relief from injection, Younger and Claridge[30] had a 24% failure rate after primary IDN excision and 43% after revision excision. In our experience, the pain relief associated with appropriate numbness is predictive of a good surgical outcome approximately 90% of the time.

## TREATMENT

Nonoperative treatment largely consists of shoe modification and insoles. Changing to a well-padded, rubber-soled shoe with a larger toe box provides more room and cushioning, augmenting or modifying forces on the forefoot. A soft metatarsal pad placed proximal to the metatarsal head relieves and redistributes the pressure as well. We prefer to use an over-the-counter metatarsal pad first, then, if not successful, a felt pad with an adhesive backing (Hapad). Patients are instructed to peel off a bit of the backing and place it in the shoe in various locations until they experience comfort and pain relief.

In the case of secondary neuralgia, when MTPJ synovitis or instability is present, a metatarsal bar, rocker sole, or splinting is helpful (eg, Budin splint or canopy toe strapping).

Corticosteroid injections can occasionally be beneficial, but adverse reactions and complications can and do occur. Injection volume should be small (no more than 1 mL total volume should be used). Larger volumes distend the tissues, causing pain. Also, large volumes bathe the surrounding tissues and put them at risk for rupture. After multiple injections, medial and lateral deviation of the adjacent MTP joints can occur from collateral ligament and intrinsic tendon damage. Sixty percent to 80% report pain relief with injection, but at 2-year follow-up, only 30% have some benefit.[31] Other complications, such as fat pad atrophy, may cause the patient to be more vulnerable to symptoms and recurrence. There also is a very small chance of aggravating symptoms with injection, possibly from trauma from the needle and local depigmentation.

Neuroma alcohol-sclerosing therapy (NAST) is reported to be a safe and effective treatment with multiple injections. Mozena and Clifford[32] reported an overall success rate of 61%. After further delineation, clinical improvement was better after 5 or more injections (74%) versus 39% with fewer than five.[32] Dockery,[33] using 4% sclerosing alcohol and 3 to 7 injections, had an 89% success rate and 82% complete resolution of symptoms. In comparison, Fanucci and colleagues,[34] using ultrasound-guided injections of 30% ethylic alcohol solution, achieved total or partial reduction in pain in 90% of patients at 10 months and a 20% to 30% reduction in mass. Temporary plantar pain related to injection occurred in 15% of patients. Overall, results vary from 60% to 94% reporting a reduction of symptoms.[32–35]

Pharmacologic treatment options beyond nonsteroidal anti-inflammatory drugs, include, but are not limited to oral vitamin B6 200 mg daily for 3 months and then 100 mg daily; tricyclic antidepressants such as imipramine (Tofranil), nortriptyline (Pamelor), desipramine (Norpramin), or amitriptyline (Elavil); and serotonin reuptake inhibitors (SSRIs) such as sertraline (Zoloft) and paroxetine (Paxil). Other antidepressants, such as venlafaxine (Effexor) or duloxetine (Cymbalta), or antiseizure medications such as gabapentin (Neurontin), pregabalin (Lyrica), topiramate (Topamax), or carbamazepine (Tegretol) have all been used.

Nonoperative treatment provides relief in most patients. In general, however, 60% to 70% of patients eventually elect to have surgical intervention. At times, this choice of intervention is chosen because of an inability or lack of desire to continue with the nonoperative treatment modalities, (ie, shoe modification). The decision to choose surgery is based on the patient's pain and dysfunction, which includes intolerance with conservative modalities.

## SURGICAL TREATMENT

If symptoms persist after conservative management, surgical excision is the most common treatment. Satisfactory results are not guaranteed, with reports of excellent or good ranging from 51% to 93%.[11,17,30,36–41]

Giannini and colleagues[11] presented the results on 60 patients using an interdigital neuroma clinical evaluation score, which includes pain, walking distance, sensitivity, and footwear requirements. They had an excellent or good outcome in 78%, fair in 19%, and poor in 3%. Of these, 62% had normal sensation and 57% could wear a fashionable conventional shoe.

Mann and Reynolds,[17] in a review of 56 patients with 76 IDNs, reported 71% asymptomatic, 9% significant improvement, 6% marginal improvement, and 14% failure. Of the satisfied patients, most, 65%, still had local plantar pain. It is also important to note that 32% reported normal sensation in the web space after documented nerve excision, which is important during the evaluation of a patient with recurrent neuroma.

Coughlin and Pinsonneault[37] reported, in 66 patients with 5.8 years of follow-up, an overall satisfaction of 85%. Major activity restrictions were rare, but 70% did report continued shoe wear modifications.

Womack and colleagues[39] reported long-term follow-up on 120 patients with an average of 5.6 years. Using the Giannini neuroma score, 51% had good to excellent results, 10% fair results, and 40% poor results. The average visual analog scale was 2.5. In addition, they found that second web space neuromas had significantly worse outcomes, which is contrary to Mann and Reynolds' previous reports.[17] They think that the reduced scores may be related to a higher rate of numbness (78%). It is clear that neuroma excision may have a long-term failure rate of 15% to 50%.[38,39,42]

When simultaneous neuromas are present in adjacent web spaces, dual excision or excision and release can be contemplated. Hort and DeOrio[43] performed excision and release on 23 patients, with a mean follow-up of 11 months. Ninety percent had minimal or no pain, 95% had no or minimal activity limitations, and 95% were completely satisfied. They also reported protective sensation to be present in all patients postoperatively, except one with preoperative neuropathy. In contrast, Benedetti and colleagues[44] did simultaneous excisions of adjacent web space neuromas in 15 patients (19 feet). At 5.7 years average follow-up, 53% had complete resolution, 31% minimal residual pain, and 2 patients (16%) had continued significant pain. After resection of adjacent web space neuromas, the tip and periungual area of the middle toe can have complete sensory loss and vascular compromise may increase the risk of frostbite in the winter.

The senior author (L.C.S.) prefers a dorsal incision for primary neuroma excision and the technique is well described in the latest version of the text, *Surgery of the Foot and Ankle*.[18] Thomson and colleagues[45] in a Cochrane database review show that there is limited evidence that dorsal incisions result in fewer symptomatic postoperative scars, with a relative risk reduction of 1.26 and a 95% confidence interval of 0.82 to 1.91. In contrast, Wilson and Kuwada[46] and Akermark and colleagues[36] support plantar incisions for improved exposure and decreased incidence of a major complication (missed neuroma).

## SURGICAL TECHNIQUE

A 3-cm dorsal incision is made within the involved web space, beginning at the top of the commissure of the web space, with the proximal extent ending at the metatarsal heads (**Fig. 1**). The incision is deepened to the metatarsal heads, maintaining midline orientation to avoid injuring the dorsal cutaneous nerves. A laminar spreader or

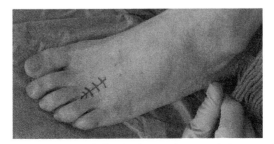

**Fig. 1.** A 3-cm dorsal incision is made beginning at the top of the commissure of the web space and extended proximal to the metatarsal head. (*Courtesy of* Stuart D. Miller, MD.)

Weitlaner retractor is placed between the metatarsal heads, putting the transverse metatarsal ligament under tension (**Fig. 2**). A neurologic Freer elevator is used to dissect the contents of the interspace. The transverse metatarsal ligament is isolated and transected. The retractor or spreader is then placed deeper between the metatarsal heads. Again, using the Freer, the common digital nerve is identified proximally and traced distally to its bifurcation. Digital pressure under the web space from the plantar aspect can be used to facilitate visualization by delivering the nerve more dorsally. There is often a significant amount of adherent bursalike tissue located dorsally between the nerve and the intermetatarsal ligament, near the bifurcation. This tissue is typically removed, but if adhesions are too great, the area maybe excised en bloc. One also makes every attempt to preserve the common and proper digital arteries lying dorsally and superficial to the involved nerve. As the nerve may be entwined with the vessel, after the nerve is divided, it is often disentangled from the vascular structures. Care must be taken to identify any accessory branches coming from the adjacent metatarsal heads, during interspace exploration. The common digital nerve is traced proximal to the metatarsal heads and transected (**Fig. 3**). It is then dissected out distally past the bifurcation and excised. Generally, we attempt to remove slightly greater than 4 cm with as little plantar fat as possible (**Fig. 4**). If a significant accessory nerve trunk passing to the common nerve is observed, the consequences of transection must be considered, such as potential retraction

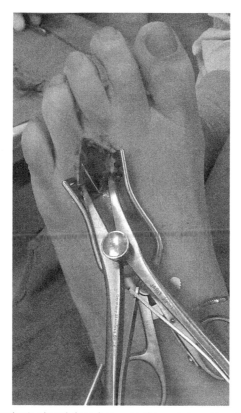

**Fig. 2.** A Lamina spreader is placed deep between the metatarsal heads. Use caution during tensioning to prevent iatrogenic metatarsal fracture. (*Courtesy of* Stuart D. Miller, MD.)

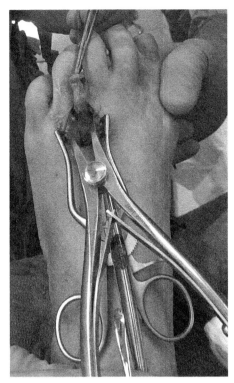

**Fig. 3.** The bifurcation and digital branches are isolated and ligated. The nerve is then delivered through the wound to allow proximal resection. Beware to identify any accessory nerve branches. (*Courtesy of* Stuart D. Miller, MD.)

underneath the metatarsal head. If the nerve trunk appears to be larger than 2 mm, rather than resecting the neuroma proximal to the metatarsal heads, the common nerve should be resected just proximal to its bifurcation, which is typically just proximal to the area of thickening. The distal portion of the nerve is removed. In this

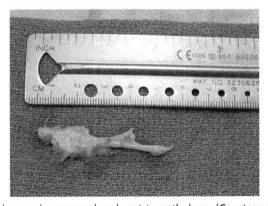

**Fig. 4.** The excised nerve is measured and sent to pathology. (*Courtesy of* Stuart D. Miller, MD.)

circumstance, the cut end should be buried by suturing it to the side of the metatarsal or one of the intrinsic muscles. Securing the cut end will help prevent the stump neuroma from falling into the weight-bearing plantar surface. In some instances, it is difficult to easily distinguish the nerve proximally, especially after multiple injections. In this situation, one can find the digital nerves distally in the toes and then dissect back to the bifurcation and proximally. If one "loses" the nerve or transects it too distally during the index procedure, it is acceptable to make a plantar incision and dissection to retrieve the nerve and manage it appropriately as indicated previously. The wound is then irrigated and the incision is closed.

The patient is placed in a postoperative stiff-soled shoe and permitted to bear weight on the heel and outside of the foot as tolerated. After 2 weeks, the patient may increase forefoot weight bearing as symptoms allow. A compressive wrap is used for 2 to 5 weeks. The patient is encouraged to work on active and passive range of motion exercises.

## SUMMARY

The initial treatment of interdigital neuralgia should consist of shoe modifications and a soft metatarsal support. If the patient continues to be symptomatic or is unable to maintain activity or shoe wear modifications, an injection of local anesthesia and steroid should be tried for diagnostic and therapeutic value. Surgical excision is indicated if this injection provides temporary relief but does not sufficiently control the pain. We believe that removal is best performed through a dorsal approach. Further research with longer-term follow-up may improve selection criteria and surgical outcomes.

## REFERENCES

1. Larson EE, Barrett SL, Battiston B, et al. Accurate nomenclature for forefoot nerve entrapment: a historical perspective. J Am Podiatr Med Assoc 2005;95(3): 298–306.
2. Civinini F. Su di un gangliare rigonfiamento della pinata del plede. Mem Chir Archiespedale 1835;4.
3. Hoadley A. Six cases of metatarsalgia. Chicago Med Rec 1893;5:32–7.
4. Tubby A. Deformities, including diseases of the bones and joints. 2nd edition. London: Mamillan; 1912.
5. Betts L. Morton's metatarsalgia: neuritis of the fourth digital nerve. Med J Aust 1940;1.
6. McElvenny R. The etiology and surgical treatment of intractable pain about the fourth metatarsophalangeal joint (Morton's toe). J Bone Joint Surg 1943;25: 675–9.
7. Gauthier G. Thomas Morton's disease: a nerve entrapment syndrome. Clin Orthop Relat Res 1979;142:90–2.
8. Graham CE, Graham DM. Morton's neuroma: a microscopic evaluation. Foot Ankle 1984;5(3):150–3.
9. Lassmann G. Morton's toe: clinical, light and electron microscopic investigations in 133 cases. Clin Orthop Relat Res 1979;142:73–84.
10. Kelikian H. Hallux valgus, allied deformities of the forefoot and metatarsalgia. Philadelphia: WB Saunders; 1965.
11. Giannini S, Bacchini P, Ceccarelli F, et al. Interdigital neuroma: clinical examination and histopathologic results in 63 cases treated with excision. Foot Ankle Int 2004;25(2):79–84.

12. Weinfeld SB, Myerson MS. Interdigital neuritis: diagnosis and treatment. J Am Acad Orthop Surg 1996;4(6):328–35.

13. Morscher E, Ulrich J, Dick W. Morton's intermetatarsal neuroma: morphology and histological substrate. Foot Ankle Int 2000;21(7):558–62.

14. Kim JY, Choi JH, Park J, et al. An anatomical study of Morton's interdigital neuroma: the relationship between the occurring site and the deep transverse metatarsal ligament (DTML). Foot Ankle Int 2007;28(9):1007–10.

15. Govsa F, Bilge O, Ozer MA. Anatomical study of the communicating branches between the medial and lateral plantar nerves. Surg Radiol Anat 2005;27(5): 377–81.

16. Levitsky KA, Alman BA, Jevsevar DS, et al. Digital nerves of the foot—anatomic variations and implications regarding the pathogenesis of interdigital neuroma. Foot Ankle 1993;14(4):208–14.

17. Mann RA, Reynolds JC. Interdigital neuroma—a critical clinical analysis. Foot Ankle 1983;3(4):238–43.

18. Schon LM, Mann RR. Diseases of the nerves. In: Coughlin MM, Mann RA, Saltzman C, editors. Surgery of the foot and ankle. Philadelphia: Mosby; 2007. p. 613–86.

19. Bradley NM, Miller WA, Evans JP. Plantar neuroma: analysis of results following surgical excision in 145 patients. South Med J 1976;69:853.

20. Thompson FM, Deland JT. Occurrence of two interdigital neuromas in one foot. Foot Ankle 1993;14(1):15–7.

21. Hauser ED. Interdigital neuroma of the foot. Surg Gynecol Obstet 1971;133(2): 265–7.

22. Graham CE, Johnson KA, Ilstrup DM. The intermetatarsal nerve: a microscopic evaluation. Foot Ankle 1981;2(3):150–2.

23. Mulder J. The causative mechanism in Morton's metatarsalgia. J Bone Joint Surg Br 1951;33:94–5.

24. Kay D, Bennett GL. Morton's neuroma. Foot Ankle Clin 2003;8(1):49–59.

25. Sharp RJ, Wade CM, Hennessy MS, et al. The role of MRI and ultrasound imaging in Morton's neuroma and the effect of size of lesion on symptoms. J Bone Joint Surg Br 2003;85(7):999–1005.

26. Kankanala G, Jain AS. The operational characteristics of ultrasonography for the diagnosis of plantar intermetatarsal neuroma. J Foot Ankle Surg 2007;46(4): 213–7.

27. Shapiro PP, Shapiro SL. Sonographic evaluation of interdigital neuromas. Foot Ankle Int 1995;16(10):604–6.

28. Bencardino J, Rosenberg ZS, Beltran J, et al. Morton's neuroma: is it always symptomatic? AJR Am J Roentgenol 2000;175(3):649–53.

29. Almeida DF, Kurokawa K, Hatanaka Y, et al. Abnormal dip phenomenon: a characteristic electrophysiological marker in interdigital neuropathy of the foot. Arq Neuropsiquiatr 2007;65(3B):771–8.

30. Younger AS, Claridge RJ. The role of diagnostic block in the management of Morton's neuroma. Can J Surg 1998;41(2):127–30.

31. Greenfield J, Rea J Jr, Ilfeld FW. Morton's interdigital neuroma. Indications for treatment by local injections versus surgery. Clin Orthop Relat Res 1984;185:142–4.

32. Mozena JD, Clifford JT. Efficacy of chemical neurolysis for the treatment of interdigital nerve compression of the foot: a retrospective study. J Am Podiatr Med Assoc 2007;97(3):203–6.

33. Dockery GL. The treatment of intermetatarsal neuromas with 4% alcohol sclerosing injections. J Foot Ankle Surg 1999;38(6):403–8.

34. Fanucci E, Masala S, Fabiano S, et al. Treatment of intermetatarsal Morton's neuroma with alcohol injection under US guide: 10-month follow-up. Eur Radiol 2004;14(3):514–8.
35. Hughes RJ, Ali K, Jones H, et al. Treatment of Morton's neuroma with alcohol injection under sonographic guidance: follow-up of 101 cases. AJR Am J Roentgenol 2007;188(6):1535–9.
36. Akermark C, Saartok T, Zuber Z. A prospective 2-year follow-up study of plantar incisions in the treatment of primary intermetatarsal neuromas (Morton's neuroma). Foot Ankle Surg 2008;14(2):67–73.
37. Coughlin MJ, Pinsonneault T. Operative treatment of interdigital neuroma. A long-term follow-up study. J Bone Joint Surg Am 2001;83(9):1321–8.
38. Friscia DA, Strom DE, Parr JW, et al. Surgical treatment for primary interdigital neuroma. Orthopedics 1991;14(6):669–72.
39. Womack JW, Richardson DR, Murphy GA, et al. Long-term evaluation of interdigital neuroma treated by surgical excision. Foot Ankle Int 2008;29(6):574–7.
40. Dereymaeker G, Schroven I, Steenwerckx A, et al. Results of excision of the interdigital nerve in the treatment of Morton's metatarsalgia. Acta Orthop Belg 1996; 62(1):22–5.
41. Karges DE. Plantar excision of primary interdigital neuromas. Foot Ankle 1988; 9(3):120–4.
42. Coughlin MJ, Schenck RC Jr, Shurnas PS, et al. Concurrent interdigital neuroma and MTP joint instability: long-term results of treatment. Foot Ankle Int 2002; 23(11):1018–25.
43. Hort KR, DeOrio JK. Adjacent interdigital nerve irritation: single incision surgical treatment. Foot Ankle Int 2002;23(11):1026–30.
44. Benedetti RS, Baxter DE, Davis PF. Clinical results of simultaneous adjacent interdigital neurectomy in the foot. Foot Ankle Int 1996;17(5):264–8.
45. Thomson CE, Gibson JN, Martin D. Interventions for the treatment of Morton's neuroma. Cochrane Database Syst Rev 2004;3:CD003118.
46. Wilson S, Kuwada GT. Retrospective study of the use of a plantar transverse incision versus a dorsal incision for excision of neuroma. J Foot Ankle Surg 1995; 34(6):537–40.

# Persistent or Recurrent Interdigital Neuromas

Samuel B. Adams Jr, MD, Paul G. Peters, MD, Lew C. Schon, MD*

**KEYWORDS**

- Recurrent • Persistent neuralgia • Interdigital neuroma
- Morton's neuroma • Morton's metatarsalgia

Recurrent or persistent symptoms following surgical neurectomy for an interdigital neuroma are not an uncommon occurrence. Persistent symptoms have been reported in 10% to 19% of patients.[1,2] This percentage can amount to a significant number of patients, considering that it has been reported that 70% to 80% of patients being treated for an interdigital neuroma eventually elect surgical treatment.[3] Beskin and Baxter,[4] in a series of 39 recurrent neuroma excisions, reported that 7 of these cases never experienced any improvement and 19 (49%) experienced only a small amount of improvement. Although most recurrences were encountered early, 18% presented greater than 4 years postoperatively. Unfortunately, there is a paucity of data to identify which patients are at risk for recurrent neuroma formation or to guide treatment once the condition manifests.

## ETIOLOGY OF PERSISTENT OR RECURRENT SYMPTOMS

Whereas the initial complaints of interdigital neuralgia are likely caused by chronic nerve compression, persistent or recurrent symptoms after attempted excision are likely because of a true neuroma. Alternatively, persistent symptoms could be the result of the incorrect initial diagnosis. The patients in Beskin and Baxter's[4] study whose symptoms never subsided most likely represent the latter, whereas patients who experience a late recurrence are most likely to have developed a true neuroma.

Wolfort and Dellon[5] postulated that a painful neuroma occurs when the proximal end of the nerve is left in a region of movement, pressure, or tension and in close proximity to the nerve growth factor that is produced by the Schwann cells of the distal fibers that are undergoing wallerian degeneration.

Mann and Reynolds[6] postulated that persistent symptoms were caused by the development of adhesions between the transected end of the common digital nerve

No funding was received for this study.
The authors have nothing to disclose.
Department of Orthopaedic Surgery, Foot and Ankle Service, Union Memorial Hospital, 3333 North Calvert Street, Suite 400, Baltimore, MD 21218, USA
* Corresponding author.
*E-mail address:* lewschon@comcast.net

Foot Ankle Clin N Am 16 (2011) 317–325
doi:10.1016/j.fcl.2011.01.003
1083-7515/11/$ – see front matter © 2011 Elsevier Inc. All rights reserved.

and adjacent structures within the weight-bearing portion of the forefoot, thereby placing traction on the nerve.

Mann[3] also suggested exploration of accessory nerves that might have been missed during the initial operation. Likewise, Amis and colleagues[7] identified plantarly directed nerve branches (PDNBs) from the common digital nerve and implicated them as a cause of recurrent symptoms. They reported on the dissection of the common digital nerves in the second and third web spaces of 5 cadaveric feet. They histologically confirmed the presence of PDNBs in every case, noting a general trend of an increased number of PDNBs branching from the distal aspect of the nerve. However, these PDNBs were also found up to 4 cm proximal to the proximal edge of the transverse metatarsal ligament, well outside the realm of a standard interdigital nerve dissection. The investigators concluded that the PDNBs could contribute to persistent symptoms after interdigital neurectomy in 2 ways. First, the PDNBs could act to tether, thereby preventing the proximal stump from retracting and keeping it in the weight-bearing portion of the forefoot and eventually developing a traction neuroma. Second, because this nerve tethering represents a small nerve bundle, injury to the PDNBs during dissection could result in traumatic neuroma formation. The investigators recommended excision of the interdigital nerve at least 3 cm proximal to the proximal edge of the transverse metatarsal ligament.

Understanding basic nerve physiology is important to understand recurrent neuromas. When a nerve is transected, there is a zone of insensitivity surrounded by a zone of hypersensitivity. This deafferentation phenomenon is a natural and possible beneficial response to a nerve transaction and usually dissipates with postoperative recovery. Anecdotally, the authors have noticed hypersensitivity in the distribution of adjacent interdigital nerves following primary neuroma surgery. It is thought that some patients are predisposed to have continued hypersensitivity. These patients may carry the diagnoses of peripheral nerve disease, fibromyalgia, or more proximal nerve compression or painful radiculopathy (the double-crush phenomenon). In these cases, there may actually be a successful resection of the primary neuroma, but the recurrent symptoms are caused by adjacent nerves becoming symptomatic.

In addition, recurrent pain may not be caused by a true plantar interdigital neuroma. It is possible that traction on the distal branches of the superficial peroneal nerve during a dorsal approach to neuroma resection can be the cause of the pain. It is often difficult for the patient to tell the difference in these 2 neuritic pain generators.

In the recurrent neuroma series by Beskin and Baxter,[4] 28 (93%) of the 30 patients were women. Although these investigators do not mention the percentage of women who underwent primary neuroma excision (196 patients), they concluded that the preponderance of women with persistent or recurrent symptoms was a representation of the population treated for primary neuromas. In addition, 30 of the 34 (88%) patients with persistent symptoms in the study by Johnson and colleagues[8] were women. The authors postulate that the high percentage of women with recurrent symptoms may also be attributed to return to certain types of shoe wear, including thin flexible soles, narrow toe box, and high heels. Women also have a higher incidence of fat pad atrophy and ligament weakness, leading to toe deformity. All these factors could lead to increased postoperative neuroma formation.

## CLINICAL PRESENTATION

Persistent or recurrent symptoms are similar to those at the time of the original presentation. Patients complain of pain in the ball of the foot, with a corresponding knot or lump sensation. Patients describe the sensation of a "wadded-up sock" underneath the ball of the foot. These symptoms are often associated with shoe wear and exacerbated by walking or running. Persistent postoperative tenderness in the affected interspace and in the area of the surrounding plantar metatarsal heads should be concerning for recurrence.[6]

The timing of recurrent symptoms is variable. Beskin and Baxter[4] reported that most recurrences were encountered within the first 12 months after surgery, but 18% presented greater than 4 years postoperatively. In addition, in the series by Johnson and colleagues,[8] reexploration occurred at an average of 33 months (range, 4–120) after the previous surgical procedure. After primary neuroma surgery, patients are advised that by 3 months they are 75% recovered and by 6 months they are 90% recovered, although recovery can take up to 2 years. However, lack of progression in recovery or increased patient frustration should raise suspicion that a recurrent or persistent neuroma is present.

## DIAGNOSIS

Reproducible tenderness in the affected interspace must be present. In general, patients with persistent or recurrent neuromas demonstrate a well-localized area of tenderness plantarly. This area is generally localized to the web spaces adjacent to the metatarsal heads. Palpation of the suspected neuroma should reproduce the patient's neuritic symptoms, such as electric-like pain. Adjacent metatarsal head tenderness could be caused by regenerating nerve innervations of the skin over the metatarsal heads.[5] Slightly more proximal tenderness, along the proximal medial or lateral metatarsal head, could represent a stump neuroma or adherence of the stump to the metatarsal. Beskin and Baxter[4] noted in their series of recurrent neuromas that the pain was localized more proximally in the metatarsal region than in the classic location for primary neuromas.

Care must be taken to rule out other causes of forefoot pain, such as synovitis, metatarsal stress fracture, avascular necrosis, plantar warts, occurrence of an interdigital neuroma in an adjacent interspace, iatrogenic nerve injury, or concomitant posterior tibial nerve compression. The physical examination should include inspection of the metatarsophalangeal joints for instability or deviation, both of which can cause traction on the adjacent nerves. Beskin and Baxter[4] identified an adjacent primary neuroma in addition to the recurrent neuroma in 5 of 30 (17%) patients. In addition, iatrogenic dorsal cutaneous nerve injury from the primary surgery should be ruled out as the source of pain.[4] Wolfort and Dellon[5] proposed that the complaints of paresthesia in the plantar aspect of the foot and toes expressed by patients with recurrent intordigital neuralgia may be related to coexisting compression of the posterior tibial nerve, and evaluation of the tarsal tunnel in this group of patients is warranted. The diagnosis of concomitant proximal compression of the posterior tibial nerve was found in 7 of 13 (54%) patients with recurrent interdigital neuromas. The complaint of numbness or pain in the affected web space is logical for interdigital neuroma, and if these complaints are more generalized to the bottom of the foot, the surgeon must entertain the diagnosis of a more proximal compression syndrome.

This vigilance must also be undertaken with the initial diagnosis of interdigital neuroma. Perhaps persistent or recurrent symptoms are actually related to the incorrect initial diagnosis. In the series by Wolfort and Dellon,[5] patients presented with recurrent pain after having multiple interdigital neuromas excised and neuromas removed from the first and fourth web spaces. Although both situations do occur, they are rare. The investigators concluded that recurrent symptoms were actually caused by true neuroma formation in the locations of resection and that perhaps the resections were done for the misdiagnosis of tarsal tunnel syndrome. Therefore, these investigators suggest considering the diagnosis of tarsal tunnel syndrome in cases of multiple interdigital neuromas or interdigital neuromas in unusual locations.

A detailed sensory examination and diagnostic injections can aid in the diagnosis. It is important that the needle for a diagnostic injection is placed plantar to the intermetatarsal ligament. Patients should experience paresthesias and pain relief in the distribution of the blocked nerve. Radiographs must be obtained to rule out osseous pathology.

## TREATMENT
### Conservative Treatment

There are few studies addressing the conservative treatment of persistent or recurrent symptoms after interdigital neuroma surgery. The therapeutic options for recurrent neuromas are the same as those for primary neuromas: shoe modification (thicker, stiffer, cushioned, wider, and increased-depth toe box), rocker-bottom shoes, and orthotics with a metatarsal pad; foot immobilization in a postoperative shoe or boot; steroid injections; typical antiinflammatories and analgesics; vitamin $B_6$; and medications to diminish nerve excitation (tricyclic antidepressants such as amitriptyline, selective serotonin reuptake inhibitors such as paroxetine, and antiepilepsy medications such as gabapentin and pregabalin). If the patient's old orthotics are used, the metatarsal pad must be moved proximally, as the old location of the metatarsal pad likely corresponds to where the nerve was already resected. Although the efficacy of these treatments is likely lower the second time around, patients may be more enthusiastic about undertaking additional conservative measures with recurrent symptoms to prevent an additional surgery. Beskin and Baxter[4] noted that in patients with persistent or recurrent symptoms, 23% had received a steroid injection before their initial surgery and 57% of the same patients received a steroid injection before revision surgery. The authors recommend that all patients be given a therapeutic injection before the initial surgery and certainly before revision surgery.

### Surgical Treatment

The success of revision surgery for persistent or recurrent symptoms after interdigital neuroma excision has been reported to be 20% to 86%.[1,3,4,6,8] Both dorsal and plantar approaches have been described for revision surgery. Traditionally, revision neurectomy through the previous dorsal incision was advised.[1,3,6] Mann[3] used a repeat dorsal approach and described symptomatic improvement in 9 of 11 recurrent neuromas. Beskin and Baxter[4] felt this exposure to be laborious in that the dissection between the metatarsals to the plantar aspect of the foot to expose the neuroma becomes increasingly difficult as the dissection proceeds in the proximal direction because of the increased diameter of the foot. Therefore, they described the plantar approach through a transverse incision located proximal to the weight-bearing area of the forefoot. Their rational for the transverse incision was the ease of exposure of additional interspaces and prevention of extension of the incision into the weight-bearing area of the forefoot. In addition, the skin creases and dermal collagen are oriented transverse to the longitudinal axis of the foot.[9] However, it is plausible that an aberrant placement of the transverse incision could limit proximal dissection for a retracted stump, and a hypertrophic scar on the plantar aspect of the foot could present a treatment challenge. These investigators retrospectively compared the traditional dorsal approach in 12 patients (14 neuromas) with the plantar approach in 18 patients (24 neuromas). Analyzing the population as a whole, 86% of patients obtained significant improvement after revision surgery. However, less than half of the patients were entirely symptom-free. About 80% of patients were unlimited in their postoperative activity, and 58% of patients (all women) experienced shoe wear restrictions. The overall results of the 2 approaches were similar, although the patients in the plantar approach group noted a more rapid, less-painful recovery time. Symptomatic hyperesthesia was also noted in 21% of the dorsal incisions. The investigators did caution against the plantar approach in patients who are known to form keloids or excessive scar tissue.

Johnson and colleagues[8] used a longitudinal plantar incision on 33 of 34 patients with persistent pain after interdigital neuroma excision. Thirty-nine specimens were sent to pathology. Of these, 26 (67%) contained elements of a primary interdigital neuroma, suggesting that the persistent pain was probably secondary to incomplete initial excision. Twenty-two (67%) patients demonstrated complete relief or marked improvement, 3 (9%) had improvement but persistent pain, and 8 (24%) had worse pain or no improvement after the reoperation. All but 1 of the 33 plantar incisions resulted in a cosmetic and functionally satisfactory scar. The 1 patient with an unsatisfactory scar had undergone a previous attempt at resection through a plantar approach. Similar to the series by Beskin and Baxter,[4] restriction of footwear after revision resection was common. Only 5 patients (15%) were able to wear any style of shoe. Twenty-two (67%) patients had minor restrictions, with high-heeled shoes being the most common restriction.

Expanding on his knowledge of painful upper extremity neuromas, Dellon[10] proposed treating recurrent interdigital neuromas through the resection of the true neuroma and implantation of the proximal stump into an intrinsic muscle of the foot. Resecting the neuroma (pain generator) and implanting the proximal nerve into a muscle that had limited excursion and was away from tension and range of motion of adjacent joints provided favorable results in the upper extremity.[11,12] In 1996, Banks and colleagues[13] reported on 16 patients with recurrent interdigital neuromas, using this technique, and implanting the proximal stump into the flexor digitorum brevis muscle. However, the results were similar to those in earlier reports not using the muscle implantation technique: 38% achieved an excellent result, 42% achieved a good result, and 20% had little improvement. Wolfort and Dellon[5] reported on 13 patients with 17 recurrent interdigital neuromas using this technique. They implanted the proximal end of the nerve into the oblique head of the adductor hallucis brevis and secured it using a 6-0 nylon suture from the epineurium to the muscle. Ten (80%) achieved an excellent result (no pain) and 3 (20%) achieved a good result. There were no problems with wound healing using this plantar approach.

### Authors' Preferred Technique

Because there is no definitive advantage in the literature of one approach over the other, the authors advise using the approach that the surgeon is most comfortable with. If there is a small dorsal incision, then it is possible that an inadequate previous resection occurred. Therefore, it is possible that repeat transection could be made through a longer dorsal incision. If the previous incision is long enough or the surgeon knows that an adequate previous resection was undertaken, then a plantar transverse incision (approximately 95% of cases) is preferred. As previously mentioned, the plantar approach allows for direct exposure of the nerve, as it lies plantar to the intermetatarsal ligament. It also allows identification of anomalous nerve branches. Finally, if there is also an adjacent web space primary neuroma, the plantar transverse incision affords both inspection of the previously operated-on web space and the ability to get to the additional web space through 1 incision. In these cases of adjacent neuromas, there is always the concern for complete vascular compromise. One of the advantages of the plantar approach is that the nerve, which lies within the perineural fat dorsal to the plantar fascia, is in this location, proximal to the convergence of the artery and vein with the nerve. Thus, revision resection carries a low incidence of vascular compromise.

The metatarsal heads are outlined. The incision is made approximately 1 cm proximal to the weight-bearing area of the involved metatarsal heads (**Fig. 1**). A small self-retaining retractor is applied to the wound. Full-thickness flaps should be developed through the subcutaneous fat and plantar fascia. Once the dissection is carried through the plantar fascia, a bulge of fatty tissue is usually evident (**Fig. 2**). The interdigital nerve lies within this fatty tissue, just dorsal to the plantar fascia and the plane of the flexor digitorum longus (FDL) tendons. In the rare case when the nerve cannot be found, the location should be reconfirmed by reexposing and applying traction to the FDL tendons while watching for toe flexion. The nerve is found between the 2 adjacent FDL tendons. Once the nerve is identified, a small curved hemostat is used to deliver the nerve (**Fig. 3**). The nerve is examined for accessory branches and transected as far proximal and distal as possible. Often a distinct bulge is not identified. The nerve should be sent for pathologic evaluation. The incision is extended medially or laterally for adjacent web space neuromas. Wound closure is performed meticulously with a 4-0 nonabsorbable suture in a vertical mattress fashion. In the plantar skin, the edges should be approximated to neutral but not everted. A compressive dressing

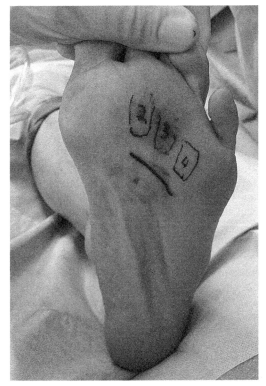

**Fig. 1.** This patient had recurrent symptoms in the third web space in addition to second web space symptoms. The second through fourth metatarsal heads were outlined. A transverse incision was made corresponding to these web spaces.

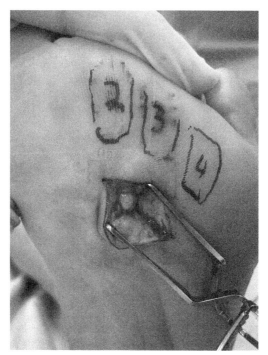

**Fig. 2.** The fatty tissue out pouching indicates that the incision has been carried deep to the plantar fascia. The interdigital nerve lies within this tissue.

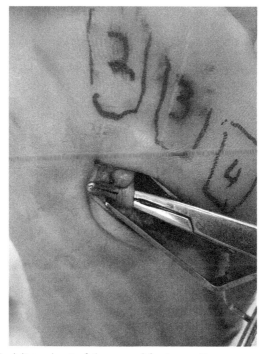

**Fig. 3.** The nerve is delivered out of the wound for transection.

and a postoperative shoe are applied in the operating room. Heel-only weight bearing is allowed immediately, and the sutures are removed at 10 to 14 days. The patient can transition to normal shoes and resume forefoot weight bearing around 3 weeks. Activity level is progressed as tolerated. Running and high-impact activities are restricted for 2 months.

The plantar approach using a longitudinal incision is performed in a similar manner. The benefit of the longitudinal incision is that the dissection can be carried proximally. This approach is especially important in a patient with recurrent symptoms who has previously had a plantar longitudinal incision. The longitudinal approach is also beneficial if nerve transposition is to be performed; it allows enough length of the nerve to be mobilized for burial. If nerve transposition is performed, a 4-0 absorbable suture is placed through the transected nerve's proximal stump. The suture is fed through a straight needle and passed through the metatarsals and through the dorsum of the foot, thereby burying the nerve in the intrinsic muscles. The suture is tied on the dorsum of the foot to help maintain the position of the nerve. The suture is cut at 10 to 14 days. Alternatively, a vein or collagen conduit can be used to guide the nerve to "nowhere". Experience with this technique is limited, but anecdotally, positive results have been achieved. If transposition is performed, the patient is to remain completely non–weight bearing for 3 weeks. In the longitudinal approach, it is important to ensure that the most distal extent of the incision is not carried into the weight-bearing area of the forefoot.

In only approximately 5% of our cases, the previous dorsal incision is used. The previous incision is extended proximally and carried through the scar tissue into the web space with careful attention to stay in the midline. A Weitlaner retractor or a small laminar spreader is used to spread the metatarsals. The previously transected inter-metatarsal ligament must be identified. It invariably reforms and must be transected. Often, the Weitlaner retractor cannot be placed until this ligament is transected. The Weitlaner retractor should also be repositioned deeper in the wound. If the metatarsal heads cannot be separated by the retractor, a portion of the transverse intermetatarsal ligament or scar tissue is still present. A neurologic Freer elevator is used to identify the common digital nerve. It is easier to start proximally in native tissue. If the nerve cannot be identified, the excision is taken proximally. Once the nerve is identified, the tip of the nerve is dissected free from the scar tissue and the nerve is cut as far proximal to the metatarsal heads as possible. Next, the ankle joint is dorsiflexed, pulling the nerve into a more proximal location. The surgical site is examined for nerve retraction. If the nerve is not retracted, a more proximal resection is undertaken. The skin is closed with interrupted sutures, and a compression dressing is applied. The patient is allowed protected weight bearing in a postoperative shoe. Sutures are removed at 10 to 14 days. The patient can transition to normal shoes around 3 weeks. Activity level is progressed as tolerated. Running and high-impact activities are restricted for 2 months.

## SUMMARY

Recurrent or persistent symptoms following surgical neurectomy for an interdigital neuroma are not an uncommon occurrence. In these patients, the presenting symptoms are often identical to the initial presentation. Recurrent or persistent symptoms must raise a suspicion for inadequate initial resection, formation of a true stump neuroma, misdiagnosis of the correct web space, adjacent web space neuroma, or tarsal tunnel syndrome. Conservative treatment is often inadequate. When surgical therapy is entertained, the preferred method is to perform revision neurectomy through a plantar transverse approach.

## REFERENCES

1. Bradley N, Miller WA, Evans JP. Plantar neuroma: analysis of results following surgical excision in 145 patients. South Med J 1976;69(7):853–4.
2. Bickel WH, Dockerty MB. Plantar neuromas, Morton's toe. Surg Gynecol Obstet 1947;84(1):111–6.
3. Mann RA. Surgery of the foot. St Louis (MO): Mosby; 1986.
4. Beskin JL, Baxter DE. Recurrent pain following interdigital neurectomy–a plantar approach. Foot Ankle 1988;9(1):34–9.
5. Wolfort SF, Dellon AL. Treatment of recurrent neuroma of the interdigital nerve by implantation of the proximal nerve into muscle in the arch of the foot. J Foot Ankle Surg 2001;40(6):404–10.
6. Mann RA, Reynolds JC. Interdigital neuroma–a critical clinical analysis. Foot Ankle 1983;3(4):238–43.
7. Amis JA, Siverhus SW, Liwnicz BH. An anatomic basis for recurrence after Morton's neuroma excision. Foot Ankle 1992;13(3):153–6.
8. Johnson JE, Johnson KA, Unni KK. Persistent pain after excision of an interdigital neuroma. Results of reoperation. J Bone Joint Surg Am 1988;70(5):651–7.
9. Courtiss EH, Longarcre JJ, Destefano GA, et al. The placement of elective skin incisions. Plast Reconstr Surg 1963;31:31–44.
10. Dellon AL. Treatment of recurrent metatarsalgia by neuroma resection and muscle implantation: case report and proposed algorithm of management for Morton's "neuroma". Microsurgery 1989;10(3):256–9.
11. Dellon AL, Mackinnon SE. Treatment of the painful neuroma by neuroma resection and muscle implantation. Plast Reconstr Surg 1986;77(3):427–38.
12. Mackinnon SE, Dellon AL. Results of treatment of recurrent dorsoradial wrist neuromas. Ann Plast Surg 1987;19(1):54–61.
13. Banks AS, Vito GR, Giorgini TL. Recurrent intermetatarsal neuroma. A follow-up study. J Am Podiatr Med Assoc 1996;86(7):299–306.

# Nerve Wrapping

Victoria R. Masear, MD

**KEYWORDS**

- Nerve wrapping • Vein wrapping of nerves
- Neurolysis • Nerve conduit

Nerve scarring can cause severe pain and dysfunction. The pain is often severe enough to significantly alter one's lifestyle. Addictive, drug-seeking behavior may result. It is not unusual for patients with nerve scarring to suffer losses of employment and interpersonal relationships.

Treatment of the scarred nerve frequently yields unpredictable results. Neurolysis may be of temporary benefit, but recurrent scarring leads to return of the neuropathic pain. The pain from extraneural scarring may result from several different mechanisms—impairment of epineural blood flow leading to nerve ischemia, circumferential scarring causing a mechanical constriction of the nerve, and adhesions prohibiting gliding of the nerve. With loss of nerve gliding, adjacent tendon and/or joint motion places traction on the nerve. A barrier wrap around the scarred nerve could be of benefit in preventing the recurrence of epineural scarring following neurolysis. The barrier would ideally be inert so as to not incite an inflammatory response, and be nondegradable. Veins fulfill both of these objectives, being biologic and nondegradable. In 1989, the author presented the first report of vein wrapping following neurolysis of scarred nerves.[1] This initial report of 24 nerve wrappings showed promising results for pain relief, and has led to many further laboratory and clinical studies. Initially autograft saphenous veins were used to wrap the scarred nerves. Because some nerves were large and/or scarred over longer distances, the need arose for a more readily available wrapping substance. Both allograft human umbilical veins (Dardik) and NeuroMend (a Bovine collagen encasement from Stryker) have been subsequently used with equal success.

The desirable qualities of a barrier nerve wrap include a substance that decreases nerve scarring, does not constrict and thus compress the nerve, and improves nerve gliding.[1,2] Weiss[3] felt that nerve wrapping could prevent fibrous tissue ingrowth at nerve repair sites and thus decrease extrinsic scarring. Nerve repair and graft sites have been wrapped with a variety of substances in an attempt to prevent suture line scarring and direct axonal growth. These substances include fat, fascia, collagen, gelatin, decalcified bone, blood vessels, cartilage, muscle, polyglactin, rubber, silicone tubing, and silastic sheeting.[3–20] Many of these materials blocked nerve

The author has nothing to disclose.
Orthopaedic Specialists of Alabama, 48 Medical Park East Drive, STE 255, Birmingham, AL 35235, USA
*E-mail address:* wobvrm@bellsouth.net

neovascularization, caused edema and fibrosis, and in some cases degraded. Silastic tubing and silastic sheeting have achieved the best success in the prevention of scar formation. These materials develop a pseudosynovial sheath with minimal host reaction and no adhesions. However, if a nerve is wrapped over a long distance with silicone or silastic, these impervious substances will prevent vascular ingrowth. Local vascularized muscle, fascia, and fat pads, as well as pedicled and free vascularized flaps have also been used to wrap scarred nerves following neurolysis.[21–23] The local materials often do not provide adequate coverage, and the flaps may be too bulky to wrap the nerve circumferentially.

## PATIENT PRESENTATION

Patients with scarred nerves usually have a history of previous surgery (often for nerve decompression), infection, or trauma (open fracture or crush injury). These patients often present with severe pain that is unrelenting, but worsens with touch or pressure over the involved nerve and with activity and nearby joint or tendon motion. Many will also have nerve dysfunction including paresthesias, numbness, dysesthesias and weakness. The history most predictive of nerve scarring as the cause of the patient's pain is one of a previous neurolysis that has provided short-term pain relief. The symptoms may have subsided for several weeks or months until recurrent scar formation causes return of the pain.

Physical examination may reveal tenderness over the involved nerve, diminished sensibility, paresthesias reproduced by joint motion or passive stretch of adjacent tendons, and positive nerve compression test. With more severe scarring or intrinsic nerve damage, motor deficits including weakness and muscular atrophy may be present.

Nerve conduction studies usually demonstrate slowing of nerve velocities in the presence of nerve scarring. Both sensory and motor latencies may be delayed. However, when scar inhibits nerve gliding and produces a traction neuropathy, without actually compressing the nerve, nerve studies may be normal.

## TREATMENT

If patients have muscular atrophy or objectively measureable loss of sensation, proceeding directly with surgical neurolysis and nerve wrapping is indicated. For other patients with suspected epineural scarring, a structured, nonoperative regimen of treatment to reduce pain should be instituted first. Nonoperative measures should include therapy to desensitize, scar mobilization, iontophoresis, and ultrasonography. Reduction of motion by splinting nearby joints can be helpful. Protective pads are used to decrease external contact with hypersensitive areas. Transcutaneous nerve stimulation (TENS), local corticosteroid injections, and regional or spinal nerve blocks can all aid in pain reduction.

Oral medications such as nonsteroidal anti-inflammatory agents can aid in pain reduction. Amitriptyline (Elavil) and anticonvulsant drugs including gabapentin (Neurontin) and pregabalin (Lyrica) are normally helpful, but can have significant side effects (especially drowsiness). Narcotic analgesics are avoided if possible because of the chronic nature of nerve scarring.

## INDICATIONS FOR NERVE WRAPPING

If nonoperative treatment fails to satisfactorily reduce the patient's pain, then decompression of the nerve and neurolysis are indicated. The primary indication for nerve wrapping is cicatrix that can both compress the nerve and cause adhesions between the nerve and surrounding tissues. The best candidates for nerve wrapping are those whose pain was previously temporarily alleviated with neurolysis. Within several weeks to months the pain can return, indicating recurrent scar formation as the cause of pain. In these patients, neurolysis to reduce adhesions and insertion of a barrier that will prevent recurrence of scarring to the nerve will likely give lasting pain relief.

An end neuroma or a neuroma in continuity are secondary indications for nerve wrapping. Wrapping the neuroma can pad the nerve to help with contact pain and prevent adhesions to the neuroma that cause pain from traction on the nerve.

## SURGICAL TECHNIQUE OF NERVE WRAPPING

A broad-spectrum antibiotic (cephalosporin) is given perioperatively. An incision is made over the region of the involved nerve. If there was a previous incision, the same incision line is opened with extension of the original incision by an additional 2 to 3 cm both proximally and distally. The involved nerve is then identified in normal, unscarred tissue both proximally and distally. The nerve is then carefully dissected free from surrounding scar throughout the length of the wound. The nerve is decompressed and gently, circumferentially neurolyzed. Care must be taken to preserve any nerve branches. To prevent devascularization of the nerve, the epineurium is left in continuity with the nerve. If there is a constricting, circumferential scar around the nerve, a longitudinal epineurotomy is performed, making sure that the epineurium is left with the nerve fascicles. However, epineurotomy is rarely necessary and should be avoided if possible, as more dissection and handling of the nerve will tend to increase the amount of postoperative pain. The length of nerve is measured, as the entire length of exposed nerve will be wrapped. Tenolysis of any adjacent, scarred tendons must also be performed.

If autograft vein is to be used for the wrapping, the greater saphenous vein is normally the vein of choice. It is easily harvested on the medial side of the lower leg and/or thigh depending on what length is needed. For example, when wrapping a tibial nerve at the level of the ankle, the length of harvested saphenous vein should be 4 to 5 times the length of exposed nerve that will be wrapped. The vein is approached just anterior to the medial malleolus and followed proximally as far as needed. The vein is suture ligated proximally and distally, any side branches are clamped with Ligaclips, and the vein is removed. The leg donor wound is then closed.

Alternatively, the saphenous vein may be removed with a vein stripper.[24] An allograft glutaraldehyde-preserved human umbilical vein (Dardik graft) has been the author's wrap of choice for scarred nerves, but is no longer clinically available. To date, a bovine collagen wrap (NeuroMend from Stryker, Kalamazoo, MI, USA) has been used as a wrapping substance for scarred nerves.

The vein or collagen is then slit longitudinally. The vein intima is placed against the nerve and the vein is spiraled around the nerve in a barber pole fashion (**Fig. 1**). A hemostat should be easily admitted between the vein and nerve at each loop to ensure that the wrap is not too snug. The vein-to-vein junctures are sutured together with 6-0 nylon sutures, using an average of 3 sutures for each complete spiral (360°). When suturing of the vein is complete, there should be no gaps in the vein junctures that expose the underlying nerve. If the diameter of the nerve is smaller than the vein, the vein can be slit longitudinally and fit sleeve-like over the nerve and sutured back longitudinally (**Fig. 2**). Because overlying skin may be thinned and friable in these patients who have often had several previous surgeries on the involved nerve, it is imperative that the wound is meticulously closed.

If a large-diameter nerve or nerve of greater length is to be wrapped, then an off-the-shelf wrapping substance is probably the best choice. NeuroMend is a Bovine

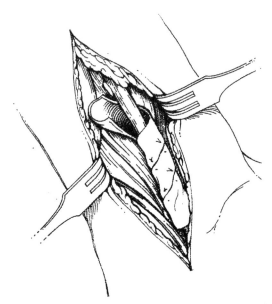

**Fig. 1.** The vein has been longitudinally slit and is then spiraled around the nerve. Vein junctures are closed with 6-0 nylon sutures. (*From* Omer GE Jr, Spinner M, Van Beeks AL, editors. Management of peripheral nerve problems. 2nd edition. Philadelphia: WB Saunders; 1998. p. 154; with permission.)

collagen encasement. The NeuroMend is self-curling. It must first be hydrated in sterile physiologic saline for 5 minutes. After hydration, it is trimmed to the appropriate length. The wrap is then uncoiled and placed around the neurolyzed nerve. The wrap automatically recoils around the nerve and maintains a self closure. If the wrap overlaps itself by about 25%, it essentially seals itself around the nerve. One 6.0–8.0 nylon suture at each end of the NeuroMend to suture the wrap to itself will ensure that it does not dislodge from the nerve (**Fig. 3**). If the NeuroMend overlaps itself by more than 25%, the excess should be trimmed to maintain the permeability of the wrap. Neuro-Mend will wrap nerves from 1.0 to 12.0 mm in diameter. For nerves with a diameter larger than 12.0 mm, 2 wraps may be sutured side by side to increase the diameter of the wrap.

## POSTOPERATIVE CARE

The lower extremity from which the saphenous vein was harvested is wrapped in a bulky bandage for 7 to 10 days. Ambulation is allowed as tolerated. Full activity level is normally achieved in the donor leg within 3 to 4 weeks.

The extremity that had neurolysis and vein wrapping is wrapped in a bulky bandage and active range-of-motion exercises are begun immediately to digits and joints. The sutures are removed within 10 to 14 days. At that time scar and tendon mobilization techniques are begun in therapy. These exercises are continued until full scar maturation is achieved in 3 to 4 months.

## OUTCOMES

Nerve wrappings for scarring have been performed on 146 nerves in 132 patients. Nineteen were wrapped with autologous saphenous or cephalic veins, and 126 with

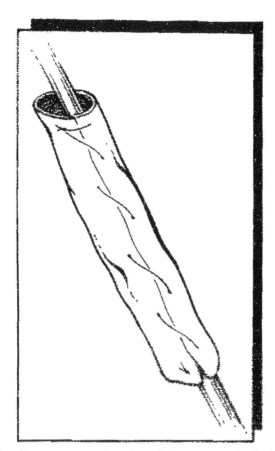

**Fig. 2.** Veins with a diameter greater than that of the nerve may be fit sleeve-like over the nerve and sutured longitudinally. The required length of vein is less than with spiraling. (*From* Omer GE Jr, Spinner M, Van Beeks AL, editors. Management of peripheral nerve problems. 2nd edition. Philadelphia: WB Saunders; 1998. p. 154; with permission.)

allograft human umbilical veins. Only one NeuroMend wrap has been used, with follow-up being too short to predict results.

A previous carpal tunnel release was the most common event leading to scarring, making the median nerve the most frequently wrapped nerve in this series. Other nerves treated with wrapping have included radial, ulnar, digital, palmar cutaneous, brachial plexus, tibial, superficial peroneal, and sciatic. The number of previous surgeries per patient prior to nerve wrapping averaged 2.4, with a range of 1 to 9.

In the first 10 nerve wrappings only the initially scarred portion of the nerve was wrapped, although the nerve dissection had been extended into healthy, unscarred territory both proximally and distally. Three of these 10 patients treated with nerve wrapping had a recurrence of pain after an initial several weeks of pain relief. Repeat exploration of these 3 nerves showed scarring at either end of the vein wrap. Their pain was relieved after extending the wrap to cover the entire length of the exposed nerve. Subsequently, all nerves were wrapped throughout the entire length of dissection.

There was a transient increase in pain and paresthesias in 6 patients. This pain subsided in 3 to 4 weeks and was thought to be caused by nerve irritation incurred

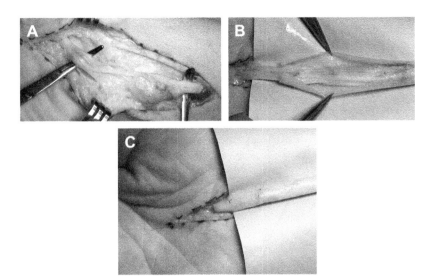

**Fig. 3.** (*A*) Following neurolysis for severe scarring of a large neuroma in continuity. (*B*) NeuroMend collagen wrap has been placed around the nerve following neuroma resection and cable grafting of unsatisfied fascicles. (*C*) 7-0 Nylon sutures have been used to tack the NeuroMend to itself, thereby preventing dislodgment.

by the dissection, and in one case a nerve wrap that may have been a little too snug. Being able to admit the tip of a small hemostat between the nerve and each loop of wrapping substance is critical.

Ten wound infections, 3 deep and 7 open sinus tracts, occurred in the group of patients with allograft vein wraps. Local debridement and removal of a small portion of the umbilical vein at the base of the wound was curative. The group of patients with autologous vein wrappings had no infections or wound problems.

Pain relief is regarded as excellent if the patient experiences only occasional pain that does not interfere with activities; good if pain is caused by strenuous activities but there is no interference with light activities and there is only an occasional use of a nonnarcotic analgesic medication; fair if there is some relief from intractable pain but splinting, TENS, and/or nonnarcotic analgesics are used on a regular basis; and none if there is no relief from the preoperative pain. Good or excellent results were achieved in 116 patients (79.6%). Of these, 58 were rated excellent and 58 good. Twenty achieved only a fair result and 10 were unimproved (poor). There was no significant difference in the results of allograft versus autograft vein wrappings.

In 17 of the 30 patients with a fair or poor result, a neuroma in continuity with intraneural scarring was found at the time of surgery. The intrinsic damage to the nerve itself was a likely contributor to their pain. Much better improvement from pain was experienced when the nerve wrapping was performed for nerve scarring only. A much more modest result was obtained when the scarred nerve also had a neuroma.

## DISCUSSION

The clinical results of pain relief have been reasonable with vein wrapping for scarred nerves.[4,24–29] The reported results for wrapping of scarred nerves have been equally good with autologous and glutaraldehyde-preserved human umbilical veins.[1,28] Treatment of the vein with glutaraldehyde diminishes its antigenicity. The human umbilical vein is tanned in a buffered 1% glutaraldehyde solution, leading to collagen cross-linking that results in a more stable and relatively nonantigenic tissue with more resistance to proteolytic digestion.[30–32] Wharton's gel and soluble proteins are then removed by subjecting the tanned veins to serial extractions with ethanol. The graft is then covered with a polyester mesh tube. The only inflammatory reaction seen with the Dardik graft has been in response to the polyester mesh.[30] When the Dardik graft is used for nerve wrapping, the polyester mesh is removed before use, and there has been a remarkable absence of scarring between the nerve/vein complex and the surrounding tissues.

Although there is no evidence of antigenicity in the glutaraldehyde-preserved vein, Ruch and colleagues[30,33] found significantly more scarring associated with a glutaraldehyde-preserved allograft than with an autograft vein. These investigators compared nerve wrapping with femoral vein autograft versus glutaraldehyde-preserved inferior vena cava allograft in Sprague-Dawley rats, and found a 10-fold increase in epineural scar thickness and a 100-fold increase in inflammatory cells with the allograft vein. There was also an increased adherence between the vein and epineurium with the allograft vein. However, there was no difference in the number of degenerating axons or in nerve function between autograft and allograft groups. The author agrees that the vein allograft adheres to the nerve. The barrier to scar formation is external to the vein wrap, between the vein and the surrounding tissues.[29] The nerve/vein complex is easily dissected from the surrounding tissues with any subsequent surgeries, and histologic studies have shown no significant scarring external to the vein wrap. There may also have been an increased host reaction in one study by Ruch and colleagues[33] because the allograft vein used was from a mature rat. The umbilical vein is less reactive because of its immature cell line.

The smooth intima of autologous veins has been shown to improve nerve gliding. Surgical procedures performed subsequent to vein wrapping of nerves have demonstrated continued gliding of the vein wrap over the ensheathed nerve.[34,35] No scarring has been found between the epineurium and the vein intima.[26,35,36] These repeat surgeries have also demonstrated minimal to no scarring between the autograft vein and surrounding tissues.[4,29,34,36,37] The vein was easily separated from both the nerve and the surrounding tissues. The vein wrap seemed to protect the nerve from both intrinsic and extrinsic scarring.[38]

Normal rat sciatic nerves that were wrapped with autologous femoral veins developed no scar tissue or inflammatory cells.[35] The wrapped nerves retained normal function, and there was no evidence of nerve compression or of contraction of the vein wrap.

In another animal model, nerves were subjected to simulated chronic compression. Half of these nerves were wrapped with veins and then compared with the other half that were not wrapped.[34] Later, histologic sections of the unwrapped nerves showed marked degeneration and surrounding scar tissue. These unwrapped specimens had fewer axons and more prevalent fibroconnective tissue. The vein wrapped nerves showed no obvious scarring. The wrapped nerves also had a greater number of axons, less degeneration, and less demyelination than the unwrapped nerves. The author has no personal experience with use of vein wrapping for the treatment of chronic nerve compression.

Tuncali and colleagues[39] wrapped nerve repair sites in rats with autologous veins to insulate the repaired nerves from adjacent arterial repairs. Two months later reexploration showed no signs of absorption or degradation of the graft and minimal adhesions between the vein-wrapped nerve and the artery. Dissection was also significantly easier in the vein-wrapped side. The study concluded that vein wraps can be used to prevent adhesions between repair sites and adjacent injured structures.

Blood vessels in vivo tend to persist indefinitely. The elastic fibers of the vein endothelium can be identified as much as 12 months later.[19] The graft architecture of the glutaraldehyde-preserved umbilical vein remains intact and it does not undergo biologic degradation.[32] The author has found these preserved vein allografts both grossly and microscopically intact as long as 13 months after nerve wrapping. Reoperations have also demonstrated no degradation of autologous vein wraps.[1,4,29,34,36–38] With time, the autologous vein wrap has even demonstrated neovascularization.[35,36,38]

Allograft veins have several advantages over autografts. Allografts do not require a secondary surgical site for harvest of a vein. Particularly with large nerves, such as the brachial plexus or sciatic nerve, or with nerves scarred over a long distance, it is difficult to obtain sufficient autologous vein. Allograft umbilical veins have no valves or branches that might leave gaps in coverage of the nerve.

Allograft veins had a higher incidence of wound problems (3 deep infections and 7 draining sinus tracts in 126 allograft wraps), as compared with no infections or wound problems in 19 autologous vein wraps. All of the wound problems were successfully treated with a local debridement and seemed to cause no adverse outcomes. With perioperative antibiotics until 48 hours postoperatively and meticulous wound closures, there have been no draining sinus tracts in the last 65 cases of allograft wraps.

Postoperative nerve conduction velocities following vein wrapping of scarred nerves have shown improvement compared with the preoperative studies.[24,26] The noted improvement was in both motor and sensory nerve conduction velocities. Electrodiagnostic analysis in an animal study showed a significantly shorter latency in scarred nerves wrapped with veins compared with scarred nerves that were not wrapped.[34]

Several clinical studies by other investigators have confirmed significant clinical improvement following vein wrapping of painful, scarred nerves.[24,25,28,40–42] Gould[25] has reported favorable results using autograft vein for nerve wrapping, while Neal and Koman[28] had a 65% success rate with neurolysis and allograft glutaraldehyde vein wrapping. Varitimidis and colleagues[24] used autologous veins to wrap scarred median and ulnar nerves, and improved pain ratings from 6 to 9 preoperatively to ratings of 2 to 6 postoperatively. These investigators also measured 2-point discrimination and documented improvement from 12 mm preoperatively to 8 mm postoperatively. Grip strength increased in their patients from 27 kg preoperatively to 38 kg postoperatively. Patients who had 2 or more failed surgeries for the ulnar nerve at the elbow who were treated by Kokkalis and colleagues[41] with autologous vein wrapping demonstrated significant pain relief, increased grip strength, and improved 2-point discrimination. Schon and colleagues[40] vein-wrapped scarred lower extremity nerves with a comparable success rate of 77% good results in 58 patients. These patient studies citing significant pain improvement following vein wrapping of scarred nerves show much better results than when the vein wrapping is used for painful neuromas.[29,43] Vein wrapping improves neuroma pain, but is more successful when combined with other procedures such as burying the neuroma in muscle and/or muscle or flap transfer for padding.

## COLLAGEN WRAPS

Stryker produces collagen wraps that can be used as nerve conduits for nerve repairs or for wrapping nerves to provide a protective environment. NeuroMend is a nonrestrictive, Type 1 bovine collagen wrap. It blocks migration of fibroblast cells, yet permits diffusion of nutrients to the nerve. NeuroMend is reabsorbed within 3 to 6 months, but any surrounding scar should be defined and matured by then. It is sized to wrap nerves varying between 1.0 and 12.0 mm in diameter. Other qualities include hypoimmunogenicity, and a rolled design that is self-curling and allows the wrap to curl over itself, thus eliminating the need for sutures except for a stay suture at each end. Contraindications to the use of NeuroMend include infection, contaminated wounds, and a history of allergic reaction to collagen or bovine products.

## SUMMARY

The addition of nerve wrapping to a neurolysis procedure has proven to be very successful in relieving the pain from scarred nerves and in preventing the recurrence of scar adhesions to the nerve. The primary indication for nerve wrapping is a nerve with adherent scar. The best predictor of success for nerve wrapping is a prior neurolysis that has given temporary pain relief. Care must be taken to ensure that the wrap is not applied too snugly around the nerve, as it may constrict. The entire length of nerve exposed during neurolysis should be wrapped to prevent extension of nerve scarring at either end of the wrap.

## EDITOR'S NOTE

We have used the commercially available collagen wraps in more than 60 cases in the past 5 years. The corrugated product described by Masear is technically easy to handle and does not kink as do the others, which also makes it attractive when used as a conduit. Our results with pain relief, to date, are excellent and comparable with the results described for vein and venous allograft. We have not experienced any wound infections or allergic reactions to the materials in our series. The convenience and lack of donor site morbidity makes these products a potentially superior option to the classic tissues described in this article. *J.S. Gould, MD.*

## REFERENCES

1. Masear VR, Tullos J, St Mary E, et al. Venous wrapping of nerves to prevent scarring. Presented at the 44th Annual Meeting of the American Society for Surgery of the Hand. Seattle (WA), September 9, 1989.
2. Sarris IK, Sotereanos DG. Vein wrapping with autologous graft for recalcitrant median nerve compression. Atlas Hand Clin 2002;7:287–93.
3. Weiss P. The technology of nerve regeneration: a review: sutureless tubulation and related methods of nerve repair. J Neurosurg 1944;1:400–50.
4. Masear VR, Colgin S. The treatment of epineural scarring with allograft vein wrapping. Hand Clin 1996;12:773–9.
5. Brunelli G, Fontata G, Jager C, et al. Chemotactic arrangement of axons inside and distal to a venous graft. J Reconstr Microsurg 1987;3:87–93.
6. Bunger O. Ueber die degenerations- und regenerations-vorgange am nerven- nach verletzungen. Beiter Pathol Anat 1891;10:321 [in German].
7. Campbell JB, Luzio J. Facial nerve repair: new surgical techniques. Trans Am Acad Opthalmol Otolaryngol 1964;68:1068–75.
8. Chiu DTW, Lovelace RE, Yu LT, et al. Comparative electrophysiologic evaluation of nerve grafts and autogenous vein grafts as nerve conduits: an experimental study. J Reconstr Microsurg 1988;4:303–9.

9. Ducker TB, Hayes GJ. A comparative study of the technique of nerve repair. Surg Forum 1967;28:443–5.
10. Ducker TB, Hayes GJ. Peripheral nerve injuries: a comparative study of the anatomical and functional results following primary nerve repair in chimpanzees. Mil Med 1968;133(4):298–302.
11. Ducker TB, Hayes GJ. Experimental improvements in the use of silastic cuff for peripheral nerve repair. J Neurosurg 1968;28:582–7.
12. Gluck T. Ueber neuroplastik auf dem wege der transplantation. Arch Klin Chir 1880;25:696 [in German].
13. Kline DG, Hayes GJ. The use of a resorbable wrapper for peripheral nerve repair. J Neurosurg 1954;21:737.
14. Lundborg G, Dahlin LB, Danielsen N, et al. Nerve regeneration in silicone chambers: influence of gap length and of distal stump components. Exp Neurol 1982; 75:61–75.
15. Molander H, Olsson Y, Engkuist O, et al. Regeneration of peripheral nerve through a polyglactin tube. Muscle Nerve 1982;5:54–7.
16. Sherren J. Some points in the surgery of the peripheral nerves. Edinb Med J 1906;20:297–332.
17. Spurling RG. The use of tantalum wire and foil in the repair of peripheral nerves. Surg Clin North Am 1943;23:1491–504.
18. Stensaas L, Bloch LM, Garcia R, et al. Snug tubular enclosures reduce extrafascicular axonal escape at peripheral nerve repair sites. Exp Neurol 1989;103:135–45.
19. Suematsu N, Atsuta Y, Hirayama T. Vein graft for repair of peripheral nerve gap. J Reconstr Microsurg 1988;4:313–8.
20. Rhoades CE, Mowery CA, Gelberman RH. Results of internal neurolysis of the median nerve for severe carpal tunnel syndrome. J Bone Joint Surg Am 1985; 67:253–6.
21. Urbaniak JR. Complications of treatment of carpal tunnel syndrome. In: Gelberman RH, editor. Operative nerve repair and reconstruction. Philadelphia: JB Lippincott; 1991. p. 967–79.
22. Botte MJ, von Schroeder HP, Abrams RA, et al. Recurrent carpal tunnel syndrome. Hand Clin 1996;12:731–43.
23. Rose EH, Norris MS, Kowalski TA, et al. Palmaris brevis turnover flap as an adjunct to internal neurolysis of the chronically scarred median nerve in recurrent carpal tunnel syndrome. J Hand Surg 1991;16:191–201.
24. Varitimidis SE, Vardakas DG, Goebel F, et al. Treatment of recurrent compressive neuropathy of peripheral nerves in the upper extremity with an autologous vein insulator. J Hand Surg 2001;26:296–302.
25. Gould JS. Treatment of the painful injured nerve in-continuity. In: Gelberman RH, editor. Operative nerve repair and reconstruction. Philadelphia: JB Lippincott; 1991. p. 1541–9.
26. Sotereanos DG, Giannakopoulos PN, Mitsionis GI, et al. Vein-graft wrapping for the treatment of recurrent compression of the median nerve. Microsurgery 1995;16:752–6.
27. Varitimidis SE, Riano F, Vardakas DG, et al. Recurrent compressive neuropathy of the median nerve at the wrist: treatment with autogenous saphenous vein wrapping. J Hand Surg 2000;25:271–5.
28. Neal B, Koman LA. Symptomatic and functional assessment of allograft umbilical vein wrapping for dystrophic median nerve dysfunction. Presented at the 49th Annual Meeting of the American Society for Surgery of the Hand. Cincinnati (OH), 1994.

29. Masear VR. Vein wrapping. In: Slutsky DJ, editor. Upper extremity nerve repair—tips and techniques: a master skills publication. Rosemont (IL): ASSH; 2008. p. 501–7.

30. Travis MJ, Harvey JH, Thornton JH, et al. Modified collagen membrane as a skin substitute: preliminary studies. J Biomed Mater Res 1975;9:285.

31. Dardik H. The second decade of experience with the umbilical vein graft for lower-limb revascularization. Cardiovasc Surg 1995;3:265–9.

32. Dardik H, Miller N, Dardik A, et al. A decade of experience with the glutaraldehyde-tanned human umbilical cord vein graft for revascularization of the lower limb. J Vasc Surg 1988;7:336–46.

33. Ruch DS, Spinner RM, Koman LA, et al. The histologic effect of barrier vein wrapping of peripheral nerves. J Reconstr Microsurg 1996;12:291–5.

34. Xu J, Varitimidis SE, Fisher KJ, et al. The effect of wrapping scarred nerves with autogenous vein graft to treat recurrent chronic nerve compression. J Hand Surg 2000;25:93–103.

35. Xu J, Sotereanos DG, Moller AR, et al. Nerve wrapping with vein grafts in a rat model: a safe technique for the treatment of recurrent chronic compressive neuropathy. J Reconstr Microsurg 1998;14:323–9.

36. Chou KH, Papadimitriou NG, Sarris I, et al. Neovascularization and other histopathologic findings in an autogenous saphenous vein wrap used for recalcitrant carpal tunnel syndrome: a case report. J Hand Surg 2003;28:262–6.

37. Vardakas DG, Varitimidis SE, Sotereanos DG. Findings of exploration of a vein-wrapped ulnar nerve: report of a case. J Hand Surg 2001;26:60–3.

38. Campbell JT, Schon LC, Burkhardt LD. Histopathologic findings in autogenous saphenous vein graft wrapping for recurrent tarsal tunnel syndrome: a case report. Foot Ankle Int 1998;19:766–9.

39. Tuncali D, Cigsar B, Talim B, et al. Insulation of simultaneous arterial and nerve repairs in the rat: the effectiveness of the autologous vein graft. Neuroanatomy 2004;3:51–3.

40. Schon LC, Lam PW, Easley ME, et al. Complex salvage procedures for severe lower extremity nerve pain. Clin Orthop 2001;391:171–80.

41. Kokkalis ZT, Sameer J, Sotereanos DG. Vein wrapping at cubital tunnel for ulnar nerve problems. J Shoulder Elbow Surg 2010;19:91–7.

42. Koman LA, Neal B, Santichen J. Management of the postoperative painful median nerve at the wrist. Orthop Trans 1994;18:765–7.

43. Masear VR, Bonatz E. Painful neuromas of the lower extremity and postneurectomy pain. In: Omer GE, Spinner M, Van Beek AL, editors. Management of peripheral nerve problems. 2nd edition. Philadelphia: WB Saunders; 1998. p. 151–6.

# Pedicle and Free Flaps for Painful Nerve

Nilesh M. Chaudhari, MD[a,*], John S. Gould, MD[a,b]

**KEYWORDS**

- Pedicled flap • Free flap • Lower extremity nerve pain
- Nerve reconstruction

Chronic nerve pain in the foot and ankle is a debilitating condition, which may develop following trauma or surgical exposure and manipulation of peripheral nerves. It may also develop from compression or traction neuritis, radiation, a stump neuroma, or a neuroma-in-continuity. The treatment of such conditions can be very difficult.

There are numerous methods of treatment described in the literature[1]: external neurolysis of the nerves[2]; rerouting of nerves by means of implantation of the neuroma stump in a muscle or bone[1–3]; excision of nonessential nerves[4]; excision and grafting of damaged nerve segments[5]; wrapping of the nerve with nonvascularized autologous (vein, fascia), allograft, or synthetic material[4–7]; or coverage of the nerve with vascularized tissue[6] whereby the nerve end is either mobilized proximally and brought into a vascularized bed, or richly vascularized tissue is brought to the painful nerve.[7–16]

## TREATMENT OF CHRONIC PAIN BY COVERAGE WITH PEDICLED OR FREE FLAPS

Kirikuta[17] initially introduced the use of pedicled flaps of greater omentum to cover the brachial plexus in patients with pain caused by radiation neuritis. Uhlschmid and Clodius[18] described microsurgical transfer of a free flap of greater omentum to cover the scarred and devascularized brachial plexus in 7 patients with chronic pain caused by radiation neuritis. Because of the successful results of pedicled and free flaps for radiation neuritis, several investigators have extended the concept to the treatment of patients with chronic pain caused by other conditions, including traction neuritis; they have also used other vascularized tissues. Millesi and colleagues[19,20] have suggested that gliding fascia is the best tissue to cover a scarred nerve. Holmberg and colleagues[13,14] described excision of the hyperesthetic area of skin, external neurolysis, and coverage of median and ulnar nerves with either pedicled groin flaps or free scapular or lateral arm flaps in 13 patients with posttraumatic neuralgia in the upper extremity. Steichen[21] advocated coverage of the scarred median nerve

The authors have nothing to disclose.
[a] Section of Foot and Ankle, Division of Orthopaedic Surgery, University of Alabama at Birmingham, 1313 13th Street, South #226, Birmingham, AL 35205, USA
[b] Division of Orthopaedic Surgery, University of South Alabama, Mobile, AL, USA
* Corresponding author.
*E-mail address:* Nilesh.Chaudhari@ortho.uab.edu

following multiple carpal tunnel release surgeries with a free omental transfer. Because of the potential morbidity of abdominal harvest of omentum, Jones and colleagues[22] described neurolysis and "wrapping" of the painful nerve with either a pedicled or free flap, consisting of either subcutaneous fat tissue or muscle.

External neurolysis and circumferential wrapping of an intact nerve with a flap may relieve the symptoms of chronic pain via 4 mechanisms. (1) A pedicled or free flap provides a more reliable blood supply than a local flap, and may promote revascularization of a devascularized segment of the nerve. (2) Wrapping the nerve with a flap may insulate the nerve from the traction forces of adjacent moving tendons. (3) The increased thickness of flap may cushion the nerve from external pressure on the overlying skin. (4) The interface between the well-vascularized flap and the nerve may result in less fibrosis and therefore allow improved longitudinal gliding of the nerve.[11,20,23]

### Surgical Technique

Indications for pedicle or free flap surgery include patients with chronic pain, who have undergone multiple previous procedures on the involved nerve, yet continue to suffer from chronic severe pain refractory to regional anesthetic blocks and pain management protocols, and require narcotic analgesics.[11]

The involved nerve should be explored, ideally, under loupe magnification. External neurolysis of the involved nerve from surrounding scar tissue is performed. Depending on the degree of scarring of the nerve, epineurectomy or interfascicular dissection may be necessary using the operating microscope. The subcutaneous fatty tissue of a fasciocutaneous flap or the muscle of a muscle flap is loosely wrapped circumferentially around the nerve.[24]

### Pedicled Flaps

Pedicled flaps may be preferred over free flaps, if available, for several reasons. These flaps do not require microvascular anastomosis. Pedicled flaps are usually based on collateral branches of main vascular axes; no major vessels need be sacrificed, as opposed to free flaps to the foot and ankle whereby end-to-end or end-to-side anastomoses to a main vessel may be necessary.

#### Distally based sural fasciocutaneous pedicled flap
The distally based sural fasciocutaneous flap is widely used for covering soft tissue defects of ankle, heel, and dorsum of the foot. The vascular inflow of the flap is provided by retrograde flow through the sural artery. The outflow is via the venae comitantes.

### Free Flaps

Free fasciocutaneous, free cutaneous, and free muscle and musculocutaneous flaps, even free fascial flaps, have all been used to cover hypersensitive nerves and cutaneous areas. Factors regarding the sites of both donor and recipient help in the decision making for the best choice of tissue. Areas requiring thin tissue coverage, such as the foot and ankle, which also have to accommodate footwear, make fasciocutaneous and muscle flaps the most desirable. The authors have used the forearm fasciocutaneous flap and muscles ranging from the rectus abdominis to the gracilis as the better functional and cosmetic choices, all of which are effective in decreasing nerve hypersensibility.

## DISCUSSION

An ischemic scarred nerve can be wrapped with omentum, fascia, subcutaneous fat, or muscle. Which one is better? Milllesi and colleagues[19,20] believe a thin flap of gliding fascia is the ideal flap for coverage of a nerve, whereas Steichen[21] advocates the omentum. Jones[11] found no difference whether the nerve is wrapped with the fatty tissue of a fasciocutaneous flap or the muscle of a muscle flap, and that both types of tissue seem to be as effective as omentum, but without potential morbidity of an abdominal harvest. Brunelli and colleagues[25] have demonstrated experimentally that if the femoral nerve is wrapped with muscle, there is 5 times more fibrosis than with omentum.

Most articles in the literature confirm positive results after either pedicled or free tissue transfer for painful nerves. However, this technique has been used mainly at forearm and hand levels,[2,8,10–13,16,26] with a few exceptions.[27–29] Coverage of painful neuromas with vascularized flaps is a two-in-one operation, whereby both the donor site and the recipient site have to be considered. The recipient site should possess patent donor vessels, with excellent perfusion in the vicinity, for establishing microvascular anastomoses of the transplanted free flap for soft tissue coverage.

The choice of the flap depends on the availability of reliably vascularized and transferable soft tissue structures in the vicinity of the of the nerve lesion. In the case of free vascularized flaps, the soft tissue is raised as a single unit based on its microvascular pedicle. The choice of the flap is also based on the ease of the operative technique (eg, favorable patient positioning, simplicity of flap raising, and the reliability of the vascular pedicle) and minimum donor site morbidity. The risks of pedicle or free flaps are flap congestion, failure of the microvascular anastomosis, flap rejection (partial or total necrosis), infection, and wound dehiscence.

## SUMMARY

Treatment of the chronic painful nerve by pedicled or free tissue transfer is a complex surgical procedure, requiring specialized microsurgical training and technique. This procedure is indicated only in patients who have had repeated failure of simpler, conventional procedures. These patients have uncontrolled pain with medical therapy and have poor soft tissue healing (repeated formation of scar with nerve entrapment). Such patients also must have no specific risk factors related to a stressful microvascular procedure (cardiac or hematological) and be able to accept possible donor site morbidities. Thus, this procedure should be reserved for recalcitrant cases of painful nerves in which simpler methods have failed.

In conclusion, patients with chronic painful peripheral nerves may be potentially salvaged by external neurolysis and circumferential wrapping of the involved segments of nerve with well-vascularized pedicled or free flaps of fascia, subcutaneous fatty tissue, omentum, or muscle; or by the replacement of superficial hypersensitive cutaneous areas and nerves with the same tissues. More studies are needed specifically in the foot and ankle to confirm the efficacy of this technique.

## REFERENCES

1. Dellon AL, Mackinnon SE. Treatment of the painful neuroma by neuroma resection and muscle implantation. Plast Reconstr Surg 1986;77:427–38.
2. Evans GR, Dellon AL. Implantation of the palmar cutaneous branch of the median nerve into the pronator quadratus for treatment of painful neuroma. J Hand Surg Am 1994;19:203–6.

3. Stahl S, Rosenberg N. Surgical treatment of painful neuroma in medial antebrachial cutaneous nerve. Ann Plast Surg 2002;48:154–8.
4. Kim J, Dellon AL. Reconstruction of a painful post-traumatic medial plantar neuroma with a bioabsorbable nerve conduit: A case report. J Foot Ankle Surg 2001;40:318–23.
5. Mackinnon SE. Wandering nerve graft technique for management of the recalcitrant painful neuroma in the hand: a case report. Microsurgery 1988;9:95–102.
6. Nelson AW. The painful neuroma: the regenerating axon versus the epineural sheath. J Surg Res 1977;23:215–21.
7. Yuksel F, Kisalaoglu E, Durak N, et al. Prevention of painful neuromas by epineural ligatures, flaps and grafts. Br J Plast Surg 1997;50:182–5.
8. Adani R, Tarallo L, Battiston B, et al. Management of neuromas in continuity of the median nerve with the pronator quadratus muscle flap. Ann Plast Surg 2002;48:35–40.
9. Krishnan KG, Pinzer T, Schackert G. Coverage of painful peripheral nerve neuromas with vascularized soft tissue: methods and results. Operat Neurosurg 2005;56:369–78.
10. Belmahi A, Amrani A, Gharib N, et al. The square pronator: an "aspirin" strip in antalgic surgery for painful neuromas of the wrist. Chir Main 2002;21:188–93 [in French].
11. Jones NF. Treatment of chronic pain by "wrapping" intact nerves with pedicle and free flaps. Hand Clin 1996;12(4):765–72.
12. Foucher G, Sammut D, Great P, et al. Indications and results of skin flaps in painful digital neuroma. J Hand Surg Br 1991;16:25–9.
13. Holmberg J, Ekerot L, Salgeback S. Flap coverage for post-traumatic nerve pain in arm. Scand J Plast Reconstr Surg 1986;20:285–8.
14. Holmberg J, Ekerot L. Post-traumatic neuralgia in the upper extremity treated with extraneural scar excision and flap cover. J Hand Surg 1993;77:427.
15. Rose J, Belsky MR, Millender LF, et al. Intrinsic muscle flaps: the treatment of painful neuromas in continuity. J Hand Surg Am 1996;21:671–4.
16. Schuind F, Van Genechten F, Denuit P, et al. Homodigital neurovascular island flaps in hand surgery: a study of sixty cases. Ann Chir Main 1985;4:306–15.
17. Kirikuta I. L'emploi du grand epiploon dans la chirurgie du sein cancereux. Presse Med 1963;71:1 [in French].
18. Uhlschmid G, Clodius L. Eine neue anwendung des frei transplantierten omuntums. Chirurgie 1978;49:714 [in German].
19. Millesi H, Rath T. Pain syndromes after nerve repair. Treatment by transplantation of gliding tissue. Meeting of International Society of Reconstructive Microsurgery. Paris (France), May, 1985.
20. Millesi H, Zoch G, Rath T. The gliding apparatus of peripheral nerve and its clinical significance. Ann Hand Surg 1990;9:87.
21. Goitz RJ, Steichen JB. Free vascularized omental transfer for the treatment of recalcitrant carpal tunnel syndrome. In: Luchetti R, Amadios P, editors. Carpal tunnel syndrome. Springer; 2000. p. 376–9. Chapter 49.
22. Jones NF, Shaw WW, Katz RG, et al. Circumferential "wrapping" of a flap around a scarred peripheral nerve for salvage of end-stage traction neuritis. J Hand Surg Am 1997;22(3):527–35.
23. Wilgis EF, Murphy R. The significance of longitudinal excursion in peripheral nerves. Hand Clin 1986;2:761.
24. Rooks MD. Coverage problems of the foot and ankle. Orthop Clin North Am 1989;20(4):723–36.

25. Brunelli GA, Brunelli F, Di Rosa F. Neurolized nerve padding in actinic lesions: omentum versus muscle use. An experimental study. Microsurgery 1988;9: 177–80.
26. Tada K, Nakashima H, Yoshida T, et al. A new treatment of painful amputation neuroma: a preliminary report. J Hand Surg Br 1987;12B:273–6.
27. Cauble WG. Painful traumatic neuroma of the vaginal cuff. J Kans Med Soc 1982; 83:10–1.
28. Satterfield VK, Jolly GP. A new method of excision of painful plantar forefoot lesion using a rotation advancement flap. J Foot Ankle Surg 1994;33:129–34.
29. Wong L. Intercostal neuromas: a treatable cause of postoperative breast pain. Ann Plast Surg 2001;46:481–4.

# Diabetic Peripheral Neuropathy

Michael S. Pinzur, MD

**KEYWORDS**

- Neuropathy • Peripheral neuropathy • Diabetes mellitus
- Lower extremity amputation

Peripheral neuropathy is defined as any disorder of the somatic or autonomic nervous systems. An appreciation of this disease entity becomes essential to orthopedic surgeons when they care for lower extremity disease or injury in the diabetic population. Whereas most types of peripheral neuropathy cause pain or impaired sensation in the extremities, when present in diabetic patients it often leads to the development of foot ulcers and infection, neuropathic (Charcot) arthropathy with subsequent deformity, and impaired immunity in healing lower extremity wounds or injury. Foot ulcers, infections, and deformity are some of the major sources of mortality and morbidity among the diabetic population. At any point in time, 3% to 4% of the diabetic population will have a foot ulcer or infection. Fifteen percent of individuals with diabetes will have a foot ulcer in their lifetime, and foot ulcers precede 85% of lower extremity amputations in diabetic patients.[1–7] In 2004 there were 71,000 lower extremity amputations in diabetic patients in the United States. Eighty-five percent were preceded by a diabetic foot ulcer.[1,8–10] Once amputated, the 2-year mortality has been reported to be as high as 36%.[11–14] These patients are at greater risk for premature death, even if they do not undergo an amputation.[11,15] An International Consensus on the Diabetic Foot estimated that in 1999, the direct cost of a diabetes-related lower extremity amputation was US$30,000 to $60,000. The long-term (3-year) cost has been estimated to be as high as $60,000 for home care and social services, and the overall cost to the United States economy has been estimated to be 4 billion dollars per year.[16,17]

## DEFINITION

Diabetic peripheral neuropathy is the most destructive type of form of peripheral neuropathy encountered by the orthopedic surgeon. It is defined as "peripheral, somatic or autonomic nerve damage attributable solely to diabetes mellitus."[18] The extent of peripheral neuropathy present in a specific patient is based on electromyography and nerve conduction studies. The threshold of peripheral neuropathy of

Michael Pinzur has no conflicts related to the subject of this article.
Department of Orthopaedic Surgery, Loyola University Health System, 2160 South First Avenue, Maywood, IL 60153, USA
E-mail address: mpinzu1@lumc.edu

Foot Ankle Clin N Am 16 (2011) 345–349
doi:10.1016/j.fcl.2011.01.002
1083-7515/11/$ – see front matter © 2011 Elsevier Inc. All rights reserved.

foot.theclinics.com

importance to the orthopedic surgeon is insensitivity to the Semmes-Weinstein 5.07 monofilament (**Fig. 1**). Failure to "feel" the 10 g of pressure applied by this nylon fiber is one of the most important risk factors for the development of diabetes-associated foot morbidity. Electrodiagnostic studies are rarely necessary for the orthopedic surgeon to assist in either diagnosis or treatment. While sensory neuropathy is the easiest to identify, its presence should alert the physician to the presence of similar levels of motor and vasomotor neuropathy.

## EPIDEMIOLOGY

The Rochester Diabetic Neuropathy Study suggested that as many as 65% of individuals with type 1 or type 2 diabetes had some evidence for peripheral neuropathy.[19] Clinical screening with the Semmes-Weinstein monofilament has detected an incidence of approximately 1 in 4.[3,5,20,21] Multiple investigators have demonstrated that the presence of clinical peripheral neuropathy is the most predictive risk factor for the development of diabetic foot ulcers (the precursor to lower extremity amputation), foot infection, and the development of Charcot foot arthropathy.[1–6,8]

## RISK FACTORS FOR THE DEVELOPMENT AND PROGRESSION OF DIABETIC PERIPHERAL NEUROPATHY

The two predictors for the development, progression, and severity of diabetic peripheral neuropathy are duration of diabetes and metabolic control. The presence of end-organ disease such as nephropathy, proliferative retinopathy, and cardiovascular disease may be a common end point of the process that leads to the development of the neuropathy.[21] The roles of excessive alcohol consumption and smoking are less clear.[22–24] Genetic factors may also play a role in the susceptibility to the development of diabetic peripheral neuropathy.

## PATHOPHYSIOLOGY

Several mechanisms have been proposed for the development of peripheral neuropathy, but none has gained widespread acceptance. There is significant support for both vascular and metabolic origins for the genesis of this common end point.

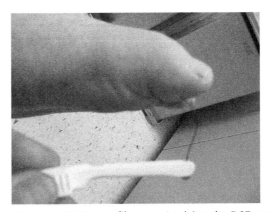

**Fig. 1.** The Semmes-Weinstein 5.07 monofilament. Applying the 5.07 monofilament to the pulps of the toes applies 10 g of pressure to the skin. Failure to perceive this amount of pressure is a key risk factor for developing all of the diabetic foot morbidities.

Investigations supporting a vascular cause have demonstrated:

- Advanced glycation of arterial vessel walls
- Basement membrane thickening
- Multifocal ischemic proximal nerve lesions
- Epineural vessel atherosclerosis
- Increased oxygen free radical activity
- Reduced endothelial nitric oxide activity
- Nerve hypoxia.

Investigations have also supported various metabolic causes:

- Accumulation of sorbitol
- Numerous studies suggesting specific enzyme deficiencies.

A bridge between these 2 proposed pathways may reside in the consistent observation of the formation of advanced glycation end products (AGEs). AGEs are formed as a result of irreversible binding of high blood levels of glucose to various proteins, producing glycated proteins or glycosylated hemoglobin that precipitate in the walls of small arterioles. This relatively slow process, associated with chronically elevated serum levels of glucose, could easily be responsible for the pathologic findings demonstrated in studies supporting both theories. There is also a substantial body of literature stating that a microvascular disease process within peripheral nerves is responsible for the peripheral nerve dysfunction.[25,26] Regardless of the pathology and etiology, it is increasingly apparent that as many as one-third of diabetic patients have evidence of some degree of peripheral nerve dysfunction.

## PAIN ASSOCIATED WITH PERIPHERAL NEUROPATHY

Whereas the orthopedic surgeon associates diabetic peripheral nephropathy with the development of diabetic foot ulcers and neuropathic (Charcot) foot arthropathy, our internal medicine and neurology colleagues are frequently confronted with the problem of pain associated with neuropathy. Experimental models would suggest that longitudinal insulin and blood sugar levels are associated with the neuropathic pain associated with diabetic peripheral neuropathy.[27,28] Of importance, numerous longitudinal observational investigations have demonstrated decreased subjective pain and rates of peripheral neuropathy–associated morbidities in patients with better diabetic control and lower longitudinal levels of hemoglobin $A_{1C}$.

Numerous classes of pharmacologic agents have been used in the attempted treatment of painful peripheral neuropathy, all with limited success. The currently available drugs with the highest patient satisfaction rates are the anticonvulsants gabapentin (Neurontin) and pregabalin (Lyrica). The second-line choice that appears to have a positive effect on peripheral nerve pain is the analgesic tramadol (Ultram). Some temporary benefit can be achieved in many patients with the use of capsaicin-containing creams and lidocaine gels. Tricyclic antidepressants, though popular in internal medicine, have had limited objective success.[29]

## ALTERNATIVE THERAPIES

Dellon[30] has demonstrated nerve conduction defects, and has suggested surgical decompression of suspected nerve entrapment at the levels of the fibular head, tarsal tunnel, and entrance into the foot at the level of the plantar fascia. Surgical decompression of multiple peripheral nerves as a treatment for painful diabetic neuropathy is a contentious issue that cannot currently be supported. Despite widespread support by proponents of this technique, no reasonable outcomes-oriented prospective trials or even reasonable retrospective case-controlled series have been conducted so as to allow recommendation of this procedure.[31]

Nonpharmacologic approaches such as transcutaneous nerve stimulation, various types of electrical stimulation, infrared, and ultrasonography have not been able to demonstrate consistent or sustained benefits.

## SUMMARY

Diabetic peripheral neuropathy likely affects up to one-third of adults with diabetes. All diabetic patients are likely to develop peripheral neuropathy if they live sufficiently long. Recognition is crucial for initiation of the preventive strategies that have been demonstrated to decrease the potential risk for the development of diabetic foot ulcers, foot infection, Charcot foot, or amputation. The mainstay of current treatment is optimal glucose and hemoglobin $A_{1C}$ control. Drug therapy has limited potential for controlling the associated pain. Alternative methods of treatment have thus far demonstrated limited success.

## REFERENCES

1. Reiber GE, Vileikyte L, Boyko EJ, et al. Causal pathways for incident lower-extremity ulcers in patients with diabetes from two settings. Diabetes Care 1999;22:157–62.
2. Apelqvist J, Agardh CD. The association between clinical risk factors and outcome of diabetic foot ulcers. Diabetes Res Clin Pract 1992;18:43–53.
3. Diabetes Control and Complications Trial Research Group (DCCT). The effect of intensive treatment of diabetes on the development and progression of long-term complications in insulin-dependent diabetes mellitus. N Engl J Med 1993;329: 977–86.
4. McNeeley MJ, Boyko EJ, Ahroni JH, et al. The independent contributions of diabetic neuropathy and vasculopathy in foot ulceration. Diabetes Care 1995; 18:216–9.
5. Rith-Najarian SJ, Stolusky T, Gohdes DM. Identifying diabetic patients at high risk for lower extremity amputation in a primary health care setting. A prospective evaluation of simple screening criteria. Diabetes Care 1992;15:1386–9.
6. Veves A, Uccioli L, Manes C, et al. Comparison of risk factors for foot problems in diabetic patients attending teaching hospital outpatient clinics in four different European states. Diabet Med 1994;11:709–13.
7. Ramsey SD, Newton K, Blough D, et al. Incidence, outcomes and cost of foot ulcers in patients with diabetes. Diabetes Care 1999;22:382–7.
8. Centers for Disease Control and Prevention Website. National diabetes fact sheet. United States, 2007. Available at: http://www.cdc.gov/diabetes/pubs/pdf/ndfs_2007.pdf. Accessed April 26, 2010.
9. Boulton AJ, Kirsner RS, Vileikyte L. Clinical practice. Neuropathic diabetic foot ulcers. N Engl J Med 2004;351:48–55.
10. American Diabetes Association Diabetes statistics. Available at: http://www.diabetes.org/diabetes-statistics.jsp. Accessed July 10, 2010.
11. Moulik PK, Mtonga R, Gill GV. Amputation and mortality in new onset diabetic foot ulcers stratified by etiology. Diabetes Care 2003;26:491–4.
12. Boyko EJ, Ahroni AH, Smith DG, et al. Increased mortality associated with diabetic foot ulcer. Diabet Med 1996;13:967–72.
13. Pinzur MS, Gottschalk F, Smith D, et al. Functional outcome of below-knee amputation in peripheral vascular insufficiency. Clin Orthop 1993;286:247–9.

14. Reiber GE, Lipsky BA, Gibbons GW. The burden of diabetic foot ulcers. Am J Surg 1998;176(Suppl 2A):5S–10S.
15. Robbins JM, Strauss G, Aron D, et al. Mortality rates and diabetic foot ulcers: is it time to communicate mortality risk to patients with diabetic foot ulceration? J Am Podiatr Med Assoc 2008;98:489–93.
16. Apelqvist J, Bakker K, van Houtum WH, et al. International consensus on the diabetic foot. Amsterdam: The International Working Group on the Diabetic Foot; 1999.
17. Larsson J, Apelqvist J, Agardh CD, et al. A decreasing incidence of major amputation in diabetic patients: a consequence of a multidisciplinary foot care team approach. International consensus on the diabetic foot. The International Working Group on the Diabetic Foot. Amsterdam 1999. Diabet Med 1995;12:770–76.
18. Proceedings of a consensus development conference on standardized measures in diabetic neuropathy. Diabetes Care 1992;15:1080–107.
19. Dyck PJ, Karnes JL, O'Brian PC, et al. The Rochester Diabetic Neuropathy Study: reassessment of tests and criteria for diagnosis and staged severity. Neurology 1992;42:1164–70.
20. Pinzur MS, Kernan-Schroeder D, Emanuele NV, et al. Development of a nurse-provided health system strategy for diabetic foot care. Foot Ankle Int 2001;22: 744–6.
21. Tesfaye S, Stevens LK, Stephenson JM, et al. Prevalence of diabetic peripheral neuropathy and its relation to glycemic control and potential risk factors. The EURODIAB IDDM complications study. Diabetologia 1996;39:1377–84.
22. Swade TF, Emanuele NV. Alcohol and diabetes. Compr Ther 1997;23:135–40.
23. Anan F, Takahashi N, Shinohara T, et al. Smoking is associated with insulin resistance and cardiovascular autonomic dysfunction in type II diabetic patients. Eur J Clin Invest 2006;36:459–65.
24. Mitchell BD, Hawthorne VM, Vinik AI. Cigarette smoking and neuropathy in diabetic patients. Diabetes Care 1990;13:434–7.
25. Tesfaye S, Harris ND, Wilson RM, et al. Exercise induced conduction velocity increment: a marker of impaired peripheral nerve blood flow in diabetic neuropathy. Diabetologia 1992;35:155–9.
26. Ram Z, Sadeh M, Walden R, et al. Vascular insufficiency quantitatively aggravates diabetic neuropathy. Arch Neurol 1991;48:1239–42.
27. Lee JH, Cox DJ, Mook DG, et al. Effect of hyperglycemia on pain threshold in alloxan-diabetic rats. Pain 1990;40:105–7.
28. Holder MD, Bolger GT. Chronic sweet intake lowers pain thresholds without changing brain mu- or delta-opiate receptors. Behav Neural Biol 1988;50:335–43.
29. Boulton AJ, Malik RA, Arezzo JC, et al. Diabetic somatic neuropathies. Diabetes Care 2004;27:1458–86.
30. Dellon AL. The four medial ankle tunnels: a critical review of perceptions of tarsal tunnel syndrome and neuropathy. Neurosurg Clin N Am 2008;19:629–48.
31. Chaudry V, Stevens JC, Kincaid J, et al. Practice advisory: utility of surgical decompression for treatment of diabetic neuropathy: report of the Therapeutics and Technology Assessment Subcommittee of the American Academy of Neurology. Neurology 2006;66:1805–8.

# Complex Regional Pain Syndrome

Ashish Shah, MD*, John S. Kirchner, MD

**KEYWORDS**

- Complex regional pain syndrome
- Impaired nervous system function
- Reflex sympathetic dystrophy • Neuropathic pain • Causalgia

Complex regional pain syndrome (CRPS) is one of the most challenging pain conditions for doctors and patients, with a natural history characterized by chronicity and relapses that can result in significant disability. It is a difficult clinical entity to diagnose and treat, and requires close follow-up to ensure that progress is being made. Early diagnosis and treatment are required to prevent a long-standing or permanent disability. Clinical features such as spontaneous pain, edema, hyperalgesia, temperature or sudomotor changes, motor function abnormality, and autonomic changes are the hallmark of this disease. The treatment of CRPS remains controversial, and includes medications, physical therapy, regional anesthesia, and neuromodulation. The levels of supportive literature are variable and sometimes limited. The main goals of CRPS treatment are the relief of pain, a decrease in morbidity, and a return to a more functional status.

In 1864 a civil war surgeon, Silas Weir Mitchell, gave the first description of this condition as "Causalgia" in soldiers sustaining nerve injuries. Since that time numerous terms have been used to describe CRPS, including reflex sympathetic dystrophy, posttraumatic dystrophy, Sudeck dystrophy, causalgia, shoulder-hand syndrome, algodystrophy, and sympathetically maintained pain.

In an attempt to reduce confusion, the International Association for the Study of Pain (IASP) used the phrase "complex regional pain syndrome (CRPS)." The word "complex" describes the different clinical presentations and the word "regional" describes the distribution of different symptoms and findings.

## CLASSIFICATION

The IASP classification system divides CRPS into two types. Overall, the clinical picture is similar in both types except for the involvement of nerve injury in the second

Division of Orthopaedic Surgery, University of Alabama at Birmingham, 1313 13th Street South, Suite 200, Birmingham, AL 35205-5327, USA
* Corresponding author.
*E-mail address:* dr.shah.ashish@gmail.com

Foot Ankle Clin N Am 16 (2011) 351–366
doi:10.1016/j.fcl.2011.03.001
1083-7515/11/$ – see front matter © 2011 Elsevier Inc. All rights reserved.

type. Another differentiating feature is that CRPS type 1 may have an orthostatic component that worsens the pain with limb dependency.

### CRPS Type 1

1. Development of pain after an initial event, that may or may not be traumatic
2. Spontaneous pain, allodynia (perception of pain from a non painful stimulus), or hyperalgesia (an exaggerated sense of pain) disproportionate to the inciting event, and not limited to the territory of a single peripheral nerve
3. History and evidence of edema, abnormality of skin blood flow, or sudomotor activity in the area of pain since the inciting event
4. No other coexisting conditions account for the degree of pain and dysfunction.

### CRPS Type 2

1. Development of pain after a nerve injury or an initial painful event
2. Spontaneous pain, allodynia, or hyperalgesia disproportionate to the inciting event, and not limited to the territory of a single peripheral nerve
3. History and evidence of edema, abnormality of skin blood flow, or sudomotor activity in the area of pain since the inciting event. No other coexisting conditions account for the degree of pain and dysfunction.

## PATHOPHYSIOLOGY

CRPS is characterized by a triad of sensory, motor, and autonomic dysfunctions, with long-standing pain and temperature differences of the affected and contralateral limb as predominant symptoms. The pathogenesis of the disorder still remains unclear. Various hypotheses have been made to reduce CRPS to a single pathophysiologic mechanism (eg, sympatho-afferent coupling)[1]; however, it has become increasingly accepted that there are different mechanisms involved. In only the past few years, it has been recognized that CRPS is not only a sympathetically mediated peripheral painful condition but also a disease of the central nervous system.[2]

The pathophysiologic mechanism of CRPS seems to be multifactorial. The mechanism contributing to CRPS differs from patient to patient, and even in the same patient it is different over time. A well-defined pathophysiology would be helpful, clinically, to design treatment protocols that address the underlying mechanisms.[3] There are number of different mechanisms most widely accepted and documented in the literature.[3]

### Central and Peripheral Sensitization

Central sensitization creates exaggerated responses to nociceptive stimuli (hyperalgesia) and converts normally nonpainful stimuli such as light touch or cold to nociceptive pathways (allodynia).[4] Affected patients also show increased wind-up to repeated stimuli-affected areas. (Wind-up is a frequency-dependent increase in the excitability of spinal cord neurons, evoked by electrical stimulation of afferent C fibers.)[5,6] CRPS-affected patients exhibit local hyperalgesia in the CRPS-affected extremity[7] along with increased mediators of peripheral sensitization (inflammatory factors, eg, substance P, bradykinin). As yet the role of sensitization in the development of CRPS has not been tested directly.

### Altered Cutaneous Innervation

Decreased C-fiber and AΔ-fiber density in the CRPS-affected areas and abnormal innervation around hair follicles and sweat glands[8] are found.

## Circulating Catecholamines

Norepinephrine levels are low in the CRPS-affected limb in comparison with the unaffected limb.[9]

## Impaired Sympathetic Nervous System Function

Wasner and colleagues[9] found that sympathetic nervous system (SNS) thermoregulatory activity was dysfunctional in CRPS patients. In their study, vasoconstriction to cold challenge was absent in patients with acute CRPS ("warm CRPS"), but it was exaggerated in patients with chronic CRPS ("cold CRPS").[10,11] As CRPS moves from the acute to the chronic state the limb turns cold, bluish in comparison to the warm, red presentation. There is pathologic interaction between sympathetic and afferent neurons within the skin.[12]

## Inflammatory Factors

Several studies and clinical trials show a relationship between CRPS and proinflammatory and anti-inflammatory factors. CRPS patients display significant increases in proinflammatory cytokines (tumor necrosis factor [TNF]-$\alpha$, interleukin [IL]-1$\beta$, IL-2, and IL-6) in different body fluids such as cerebrospinal fluids and plasma. These patients also seem to have reduced systemic levels of anti-inflammatory cytokines (IL-10) compared with controls.[13–17]

CRPS type 1 patients with hyperalgesia show much higher levels of soluble TNF-$\alpha$ receptor type 1 in plasma than CRPS patients without hyperalgesia.[14] TNF-$\alpha$ is an important cytokine, considering it has direct pronociceptive actions and induces production of other cytokines involved in inflammation, including IL-1$\beta$ and IL-6.[18]

Increased systemic levels of proinflammatory neuropeptides, including calcitonin gene–related peptide, bradykinin, and substance P,[19–22] are also found. Inflammatory factors are responsible for several features of CRPS, particularly in the acute "warm" phase. To date, no human studies have directly evaluated the role of inflammatory factors in the onset of CRPS.[3]

## Genetic Factors

There is no consistent and compelling evidence for specific genetic factors playing a role in the development of CRPS. However, the potential importance of genetic factors is suggested by the ability of some genes to influence inflammatory and other mechanisms that are believed to contribute to CRPS.[3]

de Rooij and colleagues[23] found significant involvement of HLA-B62 and HLA-DQ8 alleles with CRPS even after correcting for multiple comparisons. The involvement of HLA-B62 and HLA-DQ8 in CRPS with dystonia may indicate that these HLA loci are implicated in the susceptibility or expression of the disease. The association of TNF-$\alpha$2 allele was significantly more likely to be present in warm CRPS patients than in controls, which contributes to an exaggerated inflammatory response in these CRPS patients.[24]

## Brain Plasticity

Limited neuroimaging studies in CRPS have shown evidence of altered activity in sensory, motor (M1, supplementary motor cortex), and affective (anterior insula and anterior cingulate cortex) brain regions compared with normal limbs or healthy individuals.[14,22,25] These changes are associated with greater pain intensity and hyperalgesia, impaired tactile discrimination, and perception of sensations outside of the nerve distribution stimulated.[25–27]

There are very few studies in CRPS available to draw firm conclusions, as the brain changes on neuroimaging are nonspecific, as are changes noted in other neuropathic pain conditions.[28] Geha and colleagues[29] found that patients exhibited a disrupted relationship between white matter anisotropy and whole-brain gray matter volume. The brain exhibited atrophy of the insula, ventromedial prefrontal cortex, and nucleus accumbens, and also exhibited altered connectivity between the ventromedial prefrontal cortex and other regions. These findings have yet to be reproduced in future studies.

### Psychological Factors

Some studies showed "emotional arousal has a greater impact on pain intensity in CRPS than in non-CRPS chronic pain, possibly via associations with catecholamine release,"[30] but empirical tests to prove this hypothesis are inadequate. Further studies are required to prove the impact of psychological CRPS mechanisms.

## EPIDEMIOLOGY

CRPS can affect persons of all ages. The diagnosis of CRPS in the pediatric population was often delayed in comparison with the adult population. Sandroni and colleagues[31] conducted a population-based study in Olmsted County, and found an incidence of 5.46 per 100,000 person-years. Female to male ratio was 4:1, with median age of 46 years at onset. The upper limb was affected twice as commonly as the lower limb. In almost 46% of cases, fracture was the trigger of the event.

Allen and colleagues,[32] in a study of 134 patients (79% Caucasian), found the average time that elapsed between initial onset of symptoms and medical evaluation was 2.5 years. Patients averaged 4.8 physician consults (up to 20 consults) before being referred to a specialty center. Service-oriented occupations such as police officers and restaurant workers showed the highest incidence of CRPS, with manual laborers having the next highest incidence.

## DIAGNOSIS

CRPS classically was subdivided into 3 stages: an acute (warm) stage, an intermediate (dystrophic) stage with vasomotor changes, and finally cold (atrophic) changes. This staging system has largely been relinquished.[33]

CRPS is a clinical entity; as such, no existing laboratory study is diagnostic or pathognomonic. Its diagnosis is complex, relying on a well-directed clinical history, physical examination, radiography, and laboratory studies.

### Clinical History

Patients may or may not be able to recall a specific traumatic event that initiated their symptoms. It may be minimal injury (sprain) or severe injury (eg, nerve injury). In a study on CRPS of the lower extremity, the dominant cause was trauma (73%). Elective foot surgery accounted for the remainder of the cases (27%).[34] The most common type of trauma was a fracture (45%), whereas excision of a neuroma was the most common type of elective foot surgery. CRPS of the lower extremity is often overlooked. The key features in CRPS are spontaneous pain, hyperalgesia (pain disproportionate to a mildly noxious stimulus), allodynia (pain resulting from a normally nonnoxious stimulus), abnormal vasomotor activity, and abnormal motor activity. These clinical features persist beyond the normal time period expected for healing. Some psychological dysfunction may also be associated with CRPS.

## Pain

Patients suffering from CRPS may describe burning, squeezing, throbbing, shooting, or aching type of pain localized deep in the somatic tissue.[35] The pain usually spreads beyond the area of initial injury and can involve the entire extremity, and rarely the opposite extremity.[36] Pain can be sympathetically mediated or nonsympathetically mediated. The two types of pain frequently coexist. Pure sympathetically maintained pain is rarely seen as an isolated entity.

According to a consensus meeting of a special interest group of the IASP,[37] the diagnosis of CRPS can be made if the following criteria are fulfilled. These criteria are for clinical use.

- Preceding noxious incident without (CRPS type 1) or with a nerve lesion (CRPS type 2)
- Spontaneous pain or hyperalgesia/hyperesthesia beyond a single nerve territory and disproportionate to the inciting event
- Skin temperature, edema, motor symptoms, sudomotor abnormalities, or trophic changes present in the involved limb
- Exclusion of other possible diagnosis.

## Physical Examination

The patient may adopt a protective posture to shield the affected area from allodynia. Sometimes a stocking or glove may be worn to guard the area from mechanical stimulation.[38] In more severe forms, allodynia may prevent the clinician from examining or manipulating the affected area.

### Sympathetic dysfunction

Sympathetic dysfunction consists of vasomotor and sudomotor manifestations, which are usually intermittent and may not present on the initial physical examination. The symptoms range from a dry, warm, erythematous extremity to a cold, blue, mottled extremity. The typical signs are color, temperature changes, and hyperhidrosis. The skin temperature difference between the affected and unaffected limbs usually exceeds 1°C.[9] These findings are more prominent in the distal portion of the limb.

### Motor dysfunction

Motor dysfunction may be seen as tremor, dystonia, spasms, and loss of strength or endurance. Range of motion is decreased in CRPS. Reduced mobility may appear in the areas of dystrophy but also more centrally (eg, hip and knee). Other less common symptoms include joint swelling or stiffness. About 45% of patients also have exaggerated tendon reflexes on the affected side. Motor dysfunction is considered to be part of the pain facilitation mechanism in the absence of other neurologic abnormalities.[39] The condition may progress to brawny edema, muscle atrophy, contractures, and cyanosis.

### Trophic changes

Patients with CRPS may exhibit trophic changes including trophic/hypertophic nails, disturbance of hair growth, and atrophic skin. The skin becomes thin and subcutaneous fat disappears. The tendon sheaths and joint capsules become adherent to the underlying tendons and muscles. These changes eventually lead to joint contracture.[39]

### Complications

Complications can occur in up to 7% of cases, which include infection, ulcer, and chronic edema in dystrophic and disused limbs.[40,41] Sometimes there is an association of depression type psychological comorbidity.

## Diagnostic Tools

Besides clinical examination, several technical diagnostic tools can support the diagnosis. Nevertheless, CRPS cannot be proven by any diagnostic measure. Different diagnostic tools help to eliminate other possible causes. When vasomotor changes are dominant, vascular studies should be preformed to rule out vascular etiology. Likewise, bone or soft tissue pathology may be ruled out with magnetic resonance imaging and other radiographic studies. Electromyography and nerve conduction studies can rule out different neuropathic conditions such as peripheral neuropathies and nerve injury. These methods test only larger nerves, so smaller nerve conditions can go undetected. Infection and other rheumatologic conditions may be ruled out with generic laboratory testing including full blood count, C-reactive protein, erythrocyte sedimentation rate, antinuclear antibodies, and serum autoantibodies. A diagnosis of CRPS is made only if no other possible etiology exists to explain the constellation of signs and symptoms.

## Radiography

Plain radiographs of foot, ankle, and lower extremity (weight bearing if possible) may be able to detect osteopenia. A conventional radiograph typically shows spotty osteoporotic changes after 4 to 8 weeks.[42,43] These changes occur in only 40% of cases. The disuse osteopenia is most likely secondary to decreased use and immobilization of the involved extremity. These patients may exhibit erosions of bone cortex and a ground-glass appearance on plain radiographs.

There are 5 different patterns of bone resorption: (1) irregular resorption of metaphyseal bone, (2) subperiosteal bone resorption, (3) intercortical bone resorption, (4) endosteal bone resorption, and (5) surface erosions in subchondral and juxtachondral bone. Other endocrine disorders (eg, hyperparathyroidism, thyrotoxicosis) and metabolic disorders could have a similar radiological picture. Bone densitometry will often reflect a lowered bone mineral density and bone mineral content in affected limbs, and may be used to monitor treatment efficacy. A 3-phase bone scan may detect earlier changes, but lacks specificity.[44]

## Sweat test

Sandroni and colleagues[45] found that 62% of patients with CRPS have an abnormal quantitative sudomotor axon reflex test (QSART), showing either an increased or decreased sweat output. This test measures sweat output in response to a cholinergic challenge (acetylcholine). Quantitative sweat tests, which include the resting sweat output and sudomotor axon reflex tests, correlate with clinical signs of CRPS. A difference in sweat volume of 50% or more, or persistent sweat activity is considered abnormal.

## Thermography

Skin temperature, as a surrogate index of skin blood flow, may be used to assess vasomotor asymmetry. Infrared telethermography is considered 93% sensitive and 89% specific in the diagnosis of vasomotor disturbance.[46] An infrared thermometer is used to measure temperature changes on the affected and contralateral extremity. A difference of 1°C is considered significant, and a greater difference increases the diagnostic value of this test.[46]

Symmetric temperature findings do not exclude the diagnosis of CRPS. This test is not widely available and therefore not frequently used in the diagnosis of CRPS.

## Electromyography

Elecrodiagnostic testing may be useful to rule out any underlying nerve injury, and can be helpful in diagnosing patients with type 2 CRPS.

*Sympathetic blocks*

Diagnostic blockade of sympathetic nerves with local anesthetics helps in recognition of sympathetically mediated pain. Blockade can be helpful in patients with clinical evidence of vasomotor or sudomotor dysfunction. A block is considered successful if there is greater than 50% reduction in pain.[47,48] It can be helpful in considering these patients for permanent sympathetic block.

## CLINICAL MANAGEMENT OF CRPS
### Principles of Therapy

A multidisciplinary team approach is necessary for the optimal management of CRPS to prevent physical and psychological disabilities. The main goals of the treatment are pain control, physical rehabilitation; restoration of functionality in the patient, and preservation of limb functions.

The selection of different medications, nerve blocks, and physical therapy is guided by the severity of pain and depends on the sympathetic function status.

Psychiatric evaluation and treatment may also be beneficial in anxiety, depression, and sleep disturbance associated with CRPS.

CRPS patients often present to primary care providers for persistent pain of unclear etiology. The referral process may also begin with orthopedics or neurology and end up with a pain consultant. Timely diagnosis and validation of clinical presentation may result in a better outcome. Success can be measured in terms of pain reduction and preservation of limb function.

### Pharmacologic Treatment

*Antiepileptic drugs*

Gabapentin and pregabalin are $\gamma$-aminobutyric acid (GABA) analogues by structure. Gabapentin has been the most commonly prescribed pain medication for neuropathic pain in general; however, its efficacy as an analgesic in CRPS has not been proved. In one randomized, blinded trial in 58 patients with CRPS, gabapentin had a mild effect on pain.[49] In the largest placebo-controlled trial of gabapentin (85 of 305 patients studied) it was shown to cause a significant difference of pain reduction compared with placebo.[50]

Gilron and colleagues[51] found better analgesia was obtained with a combination of lower doses of gabapentin and morphine for neuropathic pain. Pregabalin has not been studied widely in CRPS. Its primary advantage over gabapentin is attributable to a more linear pharmacokinetic profile and twice-daily dosing.

Carbamazepine showed some good results in a very small study of 8 CRPS patients administered of 600 mg/d over 8 days in a group of 38 neuropathic pain patients.[52]

*Antidepressants*

The clinical efficacy of tricyclic antidepressants has been well documented in neuropathic pain except in CRPS. These drugs have varied anticholinergic, antiadrenergic, and cardiac side effects. Serotonin and norepinephrine reuptake inhibitors (SNRI) have been disappointing for neuropathic pain in general and specifically for CRPS. Selective serotonin reuptake inhibitors may only be considered in refractory cases after failure of tricyclic antidepressants (TCA) and SNRI in neuropathic pain and CRPS.[50]

*Nonsteroidal anti-inflammatory drugs*

Nonsteroidal anti-inflammatory drugs (NSAIDs) are commonly used to treat the inflammatory conditions of the joints and tendons, and the pain complaints of CRPS.

NSAIDs act by inhibiting cyclooxygenase and preventing the synthesis of prostaglandins, which mediate inflammation and hyperalgesia.

There have not been any consistent studies to confirm the effectiveness of NSAIDs in neuropathic pain or CRPS. Side effects such as renal failure and gastrointestinal ulceration should be monitored.

### Opioids

Opioids such as hydrocodone and oxycodone should be used only when pain has not been controlled with more conservative medications such as antidepressants. There are some favorable results demonstrating that opioids can reduce pain[53] and improve quality of life in patients with neuropathic pain.[54] However, there are no well-controlled studies demonstrating long-term improvements in neuropathic pain treated with opiates.

Much controversy exists regarding the use of opioids for treatment of chronic pain of noncancerous origin, and this is particularly true for CRPS. Side effects with opioids are common, particularly with higher doses, and include constipation, nausea, vomiting, and cognitive impairment. Opioid use can also lead to serious side effects such as respiratory depression and addiction.

### Corticosteroids

Corticosteroids have been reported to control pain, edema, and mobility in CRPS patients.[55] The anti-inflammatory effects of corticosteroids are beneficial during the initial injury response, as there is a strong inflammatory component in the early phase of CRPS. However, the risk-benefit ratio is questionable in longer courses of corticosteroids. Corticosteroids are not routinely recommended for long-term use in CRPS because of their side effects.

### Bisphosphonates

Bisphosphonates, potent inhibitors of bone resorption, are helpful in CRPS. The primary mechanism of this group is to control bone demineralization associated with CRPS, and other central and peripheral mechanisms need to be investigated in future.

Bisphosphonates (eg, pamidronate, clodronate, alendronate) have demonstrated efficacy in the treatment of CRPS in placebo-controlled[2–4,8] and small, open[1,56] studies. In placebo-controlled studies, Adami and colleagues[57] showed improvement with the use of alendronate (7.5 mg intravenously daily for 3 days), and Varenna and colleagues[58] found clodronate beneficial with a dose of 300 mg intravenously daily for 10 days. Manicourt and colleagues[59] showed better improvement in pain and edema control, pressure tolerance, and range of motion at 8 weeks with use of alendronate (40 mg daily for 8 weeks).

### Free radical scavengers

One of the theories behind the mechanism of CRPS, excessive inflammatory reaction, can lead to overproduction of free radicals. Free radical scavengers such as dimethyl sulfoxide (DMSO), N-acetylcysteine (NAC), and mannitol have been investigated for the treatment of CRPS.

Perez and colleagues[60] compared 50% DMSO with NAC in 112 patients (no placebo group), and also assessed the effect of treatment on the disability level and quality of life. The DMSO group did better overall. In a detailed study, no significant differences were found in the primary outcome measure, but warm CRPS patients did better with DMSO, whereas cold CRPS patients did better with NAC.

In another study, mannitol was found to be no better than placebo.[61]

### Vitamin C

High-dose vitamin C (antioxidant) was shown to be more beneficial than placebo in an attempt to prevent development of CRPS after wrist fracture. The frequency of CRPS with wrist fractures was 7% in patients on a daily dose of 500 mg vitamin C, compared with 22% in patients on placebo.

### Topical agents

Topical agents such as a lidocaine patch, fentanyl patch, transdermal clonidine, capsaicin, and other compound mixtures (eg, TCA, ketamine) have gained popularity for use in different neuropathic pain conditions as well as in CRPS. None of these agents have been directly studied with controlled trials for CRPS. The lidocaine patch is thought to produce pain relief by decreasing ectopic discharges within sensory afferents. The side effects of topical local anesthetics are limited, as blood concentrations obtained with local treatment are very low. Local capsaicin (an ingredient of chili peppers) induces a painful burning sensation, and is thus not tolerated well, but its efficacy has been documented in one study, in which patients were given regional blocks to tolerate high-dose capsaicin.

### N-Methyl-D-aspartate antagonists

Neuropathic pain increases the expression of N-Methyl-D-aspartate (NMDA) receptors in CRPS. Ketamine is a strong NMDA antagonist. Correll and colleagues[56] noted significant long-term benefit of an open-label infusion protocol of low intravenous doses of ketamine (10–30 mg/h) for up to 2 weeks in an inpatient setting. This concept still needs more study with fewer central nervous system agents that produce side effects.

### Medications with limited efficacy

Calcitonin was considered in the management of CRPS because of its analgesic properties, through release of β-endorphin as well as its inhibition of bone resorption. However, in most trials pertaining to calcitonin no benefits associated with its administration were detected.

Groeneweg and colleagues[62] showed marginal benefits with tadalafil (a vasodilator that inhibits phosphodiesterase-5) on a visual analog scale (VAS) in cold CRPS patients. There was no difference regarding temperature changes, activity level, and muscle strength.

Sarpogrelate hydrochloride, a selective 5-hydroxytryptamine₂ antagonist, is considered to improve peripheral blood circulation through inhibition of platelet aggregation and vasoconstriction. Ogawa and colleagues[63] did not observe differences in pain with the use of sarpogrelate in comparison with other conventional treatment measurements, except for improvement in burning pain sensation.

Wallace and colleagues[64] showed that intravenous lidocaine (a sodium channel blocker) affects pain in response to cool stimuli more than mechanical pain, and observed some effects of lidocaine on spontaneous pain.

### Regional Anesthesia

For patients whose pain is not adequately controlled by medications, regional anesthetic blocks may provide some benefit.

Patients with sympathetic dysfunction, such as mechanical allodynia with burning pain accompanied by color and temperature changes, might be good candidates for sympathetic blockade. The main aim is to provide analgesia without affecting motor functions and to involve the patient in physical and occupational therapy.

Temperature increase in the affected extremity, decreased pain, reduction in allodynia, and improvement in range of motion of the extremity without any motor or sensory blocks are indicators of response to a block.[65] Better pain response can be predicted with an increase in temperature of the limb.

### Intravenous regional block

The current available studies do not support the use of reserpine, guanethidine, ketanserin, atropine, droperidol, or lidocaine-methylprednisolone for intravenous regional block.

### Sympathetic block

Sympathetic blocks do have a role in selected patients, but not always an essential one. Several studies have been done to interrupt these pathways through local anesthetic blockade, chemical neurolysis (injection of alcohol/phenol), radiofrequency neurotomy, and surgical sympathectomy (surgical removal/electrocoagulation).

Sympathetic nerve blocks have been used for many years for CRPS, even without any supporting data. A meta-analysis of different studies comprising 1144 patients conducted by Schott[66] did not show any benefit of sympathetic blockade with anesthetic agents over placebo. AbuRahma and colleagues[67] showed effectiveness of sympathetic blockade if performed early in CRPS before central pathways set in. Two small studies (7 patients) showed increased analgesic duration of intravenous regional blockade and sympathetic block with combination of local anesthetic agents with bretylium or botulinum toxin, but further studies are needed to prove the extent of effectiveness.

Sympathectomy can be helpful to patients who are unresponsive to other treatment methods, but these patients should have at least one positive diagnostic block before being considered for sympathectomy.

Haynsworth and colleagues[68] found no analgesic differences between thermal radiofrequency and phenol neurolysis for lumbar sympathetic block, except that sympatholysis with the latter may last longer. Surgical ablation of the sympathetic chain can be performed by open or minimally invasive methods. The complications related to sympathetic blocks such as compensatory hyperhidrosis, ureteral and vascular injuries, retrograde ejaculation, and new onset of CRPS should be kept in mind.

Epidural or somatic conduction blocks of the brachial or lumbar plexus can be performed with indwelling catheters to provide sufficient pain control without affecting motor functions. This procedure can be helpful to patients who participate in physiotherapy and rehabilitation. Complications such as infection and dislodgment are associated with a catheter.

Epidural clonidine (300 μg) and intrathecal clonidine (50–75 μg) can be tried for refractory lower limb CRPS and CRPS-related dystonia, respectively. However, these drugs require further investigation.[69]

### Spinal Cord and Peripheral Nerve Stimulation

Spinal cord stimulation (SCS) was introduced as a technique for the treatment of chronic pain in the 1960s. Kemler and colleagues[70] showed significant reduction in pain intensity in the SCS/physical therapy (PT) group in comparison with the PT-only group (24/36). In a subsequent report of the first 2 years of experience with this same cohort of patients, pain relief (VAS and global perceived effect), self-report of effect, and health-related quality of life were all improved in the patients with SCS/PT.

However, at 5-year follow-up there were no statistical differences in any of the measured variables.[71] Almost 42% patients experienced at least one complication over the period of 5 years, such as failure of the pulse generator, displacement of leads, and revision of the lead generator pocket.

Recent studies do provide support for SCS as a management tool in some selected patients who respond to sympathetic blocks and a test trial of SCS.[72]

The literature does not show any favorable outcome with peripheral nerve stimulation, deep brain stimulation, or implantable spinal medication pump options for treatment of CRPS.

### Physical Therapy and Occupational Therapy

PT is one of the most important components of the treatment plan. Numerous researchers have promoted it as the first-line and cornerstone treatment for CRPS. A stepwise approach is paramount as early as possible, and ideally should be started within a few weeks of diagnosis. Goals for PT include improving pain control and increasing coping mechanisms. The PT program should be individualized for each patient based on specific impairments noted on initial evaluation. All patients should be highly motivated for PT, with mobilization and desensitization in early stages to restore a normal sensory processing pattern to the affected extremity. The first stage may be the most difficult for the patient, due to pain and phobia of having the limb manipulated and moved.

The second step is to regain flexibility and to control edema with isometric strengthening, edema-controlling devices, electrode stimulation, and manual lymphatic decongestive therapy.

The next step consists of isotonic strengthening. Progressive weight bearing should be encouraged in all patients. The goal of treatment at this stage is to increase the range of motion gradually. Aggressive passive range of motion should be avoided at this stage.

Different types of modalities such as massage, contrast baths, transcutaneous electrical nerve stimulation (TENS), and tactile desensitization should be introduced step by step depending on the recovery.

The final step in recovery includes normalization of limb function, gait training, vocational rehabilitation with work hardening and functional capacity evaluation, and workplace modification. Vocational retraining should be initiated at this time.

Each step of the PT process should be accomplished depending on severity and chronic state of the disease. Patients should be encouraged and motivated to participate. Lack of progression necessitates an aggressive intervention; on the other hand, pushing the patient beyond tolerance can aggravate the disease and hinder the recovery.

Physiotherapy consisting of a graded motor imagery program (MIP)/medical management is more effective than conventional physiotherapy/medical management. Motor imagery results are longer lasting (up to 6 months), as shown by Moseley.[73,74] The MIP consists of incorporated recognition of hand laterality, imagined hand movements, and mirror movements.

Daly and Bialocerkowski[75] did a systemic review of physiotherapy management in CRPS patients, and found that there is good-quality evidence supporting pain management PT/medical management over occupational therapy or social work/medical management.

There is no sufficient evidence supporting the effectiveness of TENS or stress-loading exercise.

The literature also supports the role of PT and cognitive-behavioral treatment in children and adolescents with CRPS. PT was shown to reduce pain and improve functions with programmed therapy.[76]

### Management of the Injured Worker

Workers with foot and ankle injuries should be evaluated thoroughly along with necessary radiologic workup. The recovery time depends on the type of injury and the number of times these patients are referred to pain clinics without any complete evaluation. It is imperative that injured workers obtain a complete musculoskeletal workup by a specialist to rule out any mechanical issues. The patients should be referred without any further delay to specialists familiar with various presentations of CRPS. In this type of patient with CRPS, delayed referral can result in delayed return to work and other issues, including litigation, which may have been avoided with appropriate care.

## SUMMARY

CRPS is a very difficult entity to manage, and the pathophysiology is multifactorial in nature. The current treatment of CRPS is mainly empirical or unclear, due to the lack of well-designed studies and the limited number of patients involved in them. Early recognition of the symptoms is important in planning a treatment algorithm that can prevent a long-standing or permanent disability. A multidisciplinary approach is essential in achieving an optimal outcome in a timely manner.

## REFERENCES

1. Roberts WJ. A hypothesis on the physiological basis for causalgia and related pains. Pain 1986;24:297–311.
2. Jänig W, Baron R. Complex regional pain syndrome is a disease of the central nervous system. Clin Auton Res 2002;12:150–64.
3. Bruehl S. An update on the pathophysiology of complex regional pain syndrome. Anesthesiology 2010;113(3):713–25.
4. Ji RR, Woolf CJ. Neuronal plasticity and signal transduction in nociceptive neurons: implications for the initiation and maintenance of pathological pain. Neurobiol Dis 2001;8:1–10.
5. Eisenberg E, Chistyakov AV, Yudashkin M, et al. Evidence for cortical hyperexcitability of the affected limb representation area in CRPS: a psychophysical and transcranial magnetic stimulation study. Pain 2005;115:219–20.
6. Sieweke N, Birklein F, Riedl B, et al. Patterns of hyperalgesia in complex regional pain syndrome. Pain 1999;80:171–7.
7. Vaneker M, Wilder-Smith OH, Schrombges P, et al. Patients initially diagnosed as "warm" or "cold" CRPS 1 show differences in central sensory processing some eight years after diagnosis: a quantitative sensory testing study. Pain 2005;115:204–11.
8. Albrecht PJ, Hines S, Eisenberg E, et al. Pathologic alterations of cutaneous innervation and vasculature in affected limbs from patients with complex regional pain syndrome. Pain 2006;120:244–66.
9. Wasner G, Schattschneider J, Heckmann K, et al. Vascular abnormalities in reflex sympathetic dystrophy (CRPS I): mechanisms and diagnostic value. Brain 2001; 124:587–99.
10. Drummond PD, Finch PM, Skipworth S, et al. Pain increases during sympathetic arousal in patients with complex regional pain syndrome. Neurology 2001;57: 1296–303.
11. Wasner G, Schattschneider J, Baron R. Skin temperature side differences— a diagnostic tool for CRPS? Pain 2002;98:19–26.
12. Baron R, Schattschneider J, Binder A, et al. Relation between sympathetic vasoconstrictor activity and pain and hyperalgesia in complex regional pain syndromes: a case-control study. Lancet 2002;359:1655–60.

13. Alexander GM, van Rijn MA, van Hilten JJ, et al. Changes in cerebrospinal fluid levels of pro- inflammatory cytokines in CRPS. Pain 2005;116:213–9.
14. Maihöfner C, Handwerker HO, Neundörfer B, et al. Mechanical hyperalgesia in complex regional pain syndrome: a role for TNF-alpha? Neurology 2005;65:311–3.
15. Uçeyler N, Eberle T, Rolke R, et al. Differential expression patterns of cytokines in complex regional pain syndrome. Pain 2007;132:14–5.
16. Wesseldijk F, Huygen FJ, Heijmans-Antonissen C, et al. Six years follow- up of the levels of TNF-alpha and IL-6 in patients with complex regional pain syndrome type 1. Mediators Inflamm 2008;2008:469439.
17. Wesseldijk F, Huygen FJ, Heijmans-Antonissen C, et al. Tumor necrosis factor-alpha and interleukin-6 are not correlated with the characteristics of complex regional pain syndrome type 1 in 66 patients. Eur J Pain 2008;12:716–21.
18. Sommers C, Kress M. Recent findings on how proinflammatory cytokines cause pain: peripheral mechanisms in inflammatory and neuropathic hyperalgesia. Neurosci Lett 2004;361:184–7.
19. Birklein F, Schmelz M, Schifter S, et al. The important role of neuropeptides in complex regional pain syndrome. Neurology 2001;57:2179–84.
20. Blair SJ, Chinthagada M, Hoppenstehdt D, et al. Role of neuropeptides in pathogenesis of reflex sympathetic dystrophy. Acta Orthop Belg 1998;64:448–51.
21. Schinkel C, Gaertner A, Zaspel J, et al. Inflammatory mediators are altered in the acute phase of posttraumatic complex regional pain syndrome. Clin J Pain 2006; 22:235–9.
22. Maihöfner C, Baron R, DeCol R, et al. The motor system shows adaptive changes in complex regional pain syndrome. Brain 2007;130:2671–87.
23. de Rooij AM, Florencia Gosso M, Haasnoot GW, et al. HLA-B62 and HLA-DQ8 are associated with complex regional pain syndrome with fixed dystonia. Pain 2009; 145:82–5.
24. Vaneker M, van der Laan L, Allebes WA, et al. Genetic factors associated with complex regional pain syndrome I: HLA DRB and TNF alpha promoter gene polymorphism. Disabil Med 2002;2:69–74.
25. Maihöfner C, Handwerker HO, Birklein F. Functional imaging of allodynia in complex regional pain syndrome. Neurology 2006;66:711–7.
26. Pleger B, Ragert P, Schwenkreis P, et al. Patterns of cortical reorganization parallel impaired tactile discrimination and pain intensity in complex regional pain syndrome. Neuroimage 2006;32:503–10.
27. Maihöfner C, Neundörfer B, Birklein F, et al. Mislocalization of tactile stimulation in patients with complex regional pain syndrome. J Neurol 2006;253:772–9.
28. Moisset X, Bouhassira D. Brain imaging of neuropathic pain. Neuroimage 2007; 37(Suppl 1):S80–8.
29. Geha PY, Baliki MN, Harden RN, et al. The brain in chronic CRPS pain: abnormal gray-white matter interactions in emotional and autonomic regions. Neuron 2008; 60:570–81.
30. Bruehl S, Husfeldt B, Lubenow T, et al. Psychological differences between reflex sympathetic dystrophy and non-RSD chronic pain patients. Pain 1996;67:107–14.
31. Sandroni P, Benrud-Larson LM, McClelland RL, et al. Complex regional pain syndrome type I: incidence and prevalence in Olmsted County, a population based study. Pain 2003;103:199–207.
32. Allen G, Galer BS, Schwartz L. Epidemiology of complex regional pain syndrome: a retrospective chart review of 134 patients. Pain 1999;80:539–44.
33. Bruehl S, Harden RN, Galer BS, et al. Complex regional pain syndrome: are there distinct subtypes and sequential stages of the syndrome? Pain 2002;95:119–24.

34. Anderson DJ, Fallat LM. Complex regional pain syndrome of the lower extremity: a retrospective study of 33 patients. J Foot Ankle Surg 1999;38(6):381–7.
35. Raja SN, Grabow TS. Complex regional pain syndrome I (reflex sympathetic dystrophy). Anesthesiology 2002;96:1254–60.
36. Karacan I, Aydin T, Ozaras N. Bone loss in the contralateral asymptomatic hand in patients with complex regional pain syndrome type 1. J Bone Miner Metab 2004;22:44–7.
37. Wilson PR. Taxonomy. Newsletter of the IASP special interest group on pain and the sympathetic nervous system. September, 2004. p. 4–6.
38. Rho RH, Brewer RP, Lamer TJ, et al. Complex regional pain syndrome. Mayo Clin Proc 2002;77(2):174–80.
39. Birklein F, Handwerker HO. Complex regional pain syndrome: how to resolve the complexity? Pain 2001;94:1–6.
40. van der Laan L, Veldman PH, Goris RJ. Severe complications of reflex sympathetic dystrophy: infection, ulcers, chronic edema, dystonia, and myoclonus. Arch Phys Med Rehabil 1998;79:424–9.
41. Bruehl S, Carlson CR. Predisposing psychological factors in the development of reflex sympathetic dystrophy. A review of the empirical evidence. Clin J Pain 1992;8:287–99.
42. Veldman PH, Reynen HM, Arntz IE, et al. Signs and symptoms of reflex sympathetic dystrophy: prospective study of 829 patients. Lancet 1993;342:1012–6.
43. Genant HK, Kozin F, Bekerman C, et al. The reflex sympathetic dystrophy syndrome. A comprehensive analysis using fine-detail radiography, photon absorptiometry, and bone and joint scintigraphy. Radiology 1975;117(1):21–32.
44. Koman LA. Current status of noninvasive techniques in the diagnosis of upper extremity disorders. Part I. Evaluation of vascular competency. Instr Course Lect 1983;32:61–76.
45. Sandroni P, Low PA, Ferrer T, et al. Complex regional pain syndrome I (CRPS I): prospective study and laboratory evaluation. Clin J Pain 1998;14(4):282–9.
46. Gulevich SJ, Conwell TD, Lane J, et al. Stress infrared telethermography is useful in the diagnosis of complex regional pain syndrome, type I (formerly reflex sympathetic dystrophy). Clin J Pain 1997;13:50–9.
47. Price DD, Long S, Wilsey B, et al. Analysis of peak magnitude and duration of analgesia produced by local anesthetics injected into sympathetic ganglia of complex regional pain syndrome patients. Clin J Pain 1998;14:216–26.
48. Backonja MM, Serra J. Pharmacologic management part 2: lesser-studied neuropathic pain diseases. Pain Med 2004;5(Suppl 1):S48–59.
49. van de Vusse AC, Stomp-van den Berg SG, Kessels AH, et al. Randomised controlled trial of gabapentin in complex regional pain syndrome type 1 [ISRCTN84121379]. BMC Neurol 2004;4:13.
50. Serpell MG. Gabapentin in neuropathic pain syndromes: a randomised, double-blind, placebo-controlled trial. Pain 2002;99:557–66.
51. Gilron I, Bailey JM, Tu D, et al. Morphine, gabapentin, or their combination for neuropathic pain. N Engl J Med 2005;352:1324–34.
52. Harke H, Gretenkort P, Ladleif HU, et al. The response of neuropathic pain and pain in complex regional pain syndrome I to carbamazepine and sustained-release morphine in patients pretreated with spinal cord stimulation: a double-blinded randomized study. Anesth Analg 2001;92(2):488–95.
53. Watson CP, Babul N. Efficacy of oxycodone in neuropathic pain: a randomized trial in postherpetic neuralgia. Neurology 1998;50:1837–41.

54. Watson CP, Moulin D, Watt-Watson J, et al. Controlled-release oxycodone relieves neuropathic pain: a randomized controlled trial in painful diabetic neuropathy. Pain 2003;105:71–8.
55. Kingery WS. A critical review of controlled clinical trials for peripheral neuropathic pain and complex regional pain syndromes. Pain 1997;73:123–39.
56. Correll GE, Maleki J, Gracely EJ, et al. Subanesthetic ketamine infusion therapy: a retrospective analysis of a novel therapeutic approach to complex regional pain syndrome. Pain Med 2004;5:263–75.
57. Adami S, Fossaluzza V, Gatti D, et al. Bisphosphonate therapy of reflex sympathetic dystrophy syndrome. Ann Rheum Dis 1997;56:201–4.
58. Varenna M, Zucchi F, Ghiringhelli D, et al. Intravenous clodronate in the treatment of reflex sympathetic dystrophy syndrome. A randomized, double blind, placebo controlled study. J Rheumatol 2000;27:1477–83.
59. Manicourt DH, Brasseur JP, Boutsen Y, et al. Role of alendronate in therapy for posttraumatic complex regional pain syndrome type 1 of the lower extremity. Arthritis Rheum 2004;50:3690–7.
60. Perez RS, Zuurmond WW, Bezemer PD, et al. The treatment of complex regional pain syndrome type I with free radical scavengers: a randomized controlled study. Pain 2003;102(3):297–307.
61. Perez RS, Pragt E, Geurts J, et al. Treatment of patients with complex regional pain syndrome type I with mannitol: a prospective, randomized, placebo-controlled, double-blinded study. J Pain 2008;9(8):678–86.
62. Groeneweg G, Huygen FJ, Niehof SP, et al. Effects of tadalafil on blood flow, pain, and function in chronic cold complex regional pain syndrome: a randomized controlled trial. BMC Musculoskelet Disord 2008;9:143.
63. Ogawa S, Suzuki H, Shiotani M, et al. A randomized clinical trial of sarpogrelate hydrochloride for neuropathic pain in patients with post-herpetic neuralgia and reflex sympathetic dystrophy. Pain Clinic 1998;11:125–32.
64. Wallace MS, Ridgeway BM, Leung AY, et al. Concentration-effect relationship of intravenous lidocaine on the allodynia of complex regional pain syndrome types I and II. Anesthesiology 2000;92:75–83.
65. Tran KM, Frank SM, Raja SN, et al. Lumbar sympathetic block for sympathetically maintained pain: changes in cutaneous temperatures and pain perception. Anesth Analg 2000;90:1396–401.
66. Schott GD. Interrupting the sympathetic outflow in causalgia and reflex sympathetic dystrophy. BMJ 1998;316:792–3.
67. AbuRahma AF, Robinson PA, Powell M, et al. Sympathectomy for reflex sympathetic dystrophy: factors affecting outcome. Ann Vasc Surg 1994;8(4):372–9.
68. Haynsworth RF, Noe CE. Percutaneous lumbar sympathectomy: a comparison of radiofrequency denervation versus phenol neurolysis. Anesthesiology 1991;74:459–63.
69. Rauck RL, Eisenach JC, Jackson K, et al. Epidural clonidine treatment for refractory reflex sympathetic dystrophy. Anesthesiology 1993;79:1163–9.
70. Kemler MA, De Vet HC, Barendse GA, et al. The effect of spinal cord stimulation in patients with chronic reflex sympathetic dystrophy; two years' follow-up of the randomized controlled trial. Ann Neurol 2004;55:13–8.
71. Kemler MA, De Vet HC, Barendse GA, et al. Effect of spinal cord stimulation for chronic complex regional pain syndrome type I: five-year final follow-up of patients in a randomized controlled trial. J Neurosurg 2008;108:292–8.
72. Nelson DV, Stacey BR. Interventional therapies in the management of complex regional pain syndrome. Clin J Pain 2006;22(5):438–42.

73. Moseley GL. Graded motor imagery is effective for long-standing complex regional pain syndrome: a randomised controlled trial. Pain 2004;108:192–8.
74. Moseley GL. Is successful rehabilitation of complex regional pain syndrome due to sustained attention to the affected limb? A randomised clinical trial. Pain 2005; 114:54–61.
75. Daly AE, Bialocerkowski AE. Does evidence support physiotherapy management of adult complex regional pain syndrome type one? A systematic review. Eur J Pain 2009;13(4):339–53.
76. Lee BH, Scharff L, Sethna NF, et al. Physical therapy and cognitive-behavioral treatment for complex regional pain syndromes. J Pediatr 2002;141(1):135–40.

# Index

Note: Page numbers of article titles are in **boldface** type.

Foot Ankle Clin N Am 16 (2011) 367–373
doi:10.1016/S1083-7515(11)00037-4
1083-7515/11/$ – see front matter © 2011 Elsevier Inc. All rights reserved.

# *Moving?*

## *Make sure your subscription moves with you!*

To notify us of your new address, find your **Clinics Account Number** (located on your mailing label above your name), and contact customer service at:

Email: **journalscustomerservice-usa@elsevier.com**

**800-654-2452** (subscribers in the U.S. & Canada)
**314-447-8871** (subscribers outside of the U.S. & Canada)

Fax number: **314-447-8029**

**Elsevier Health Sciences Division
Subscription Customer Service
3251 Riverport Lane
Maryland Heights, MO 63043**

*To ensure uninterrupted delivery of your subscription, please notify us at least 4 weeks in advance of move.

Printed and bound by CPI Group (UK) Ltd, Croydon, CR0 4YY

03/10/2024

01040455-0014